Easy Calo & Fitness Guide

MW01286463

By Helena Schaar

The easiest calorie counter ever! Alphabetical listings for fast and easy calorie counts. All the favorite foods, fast food restaurants, and beverages. Contains about 3,500 listings. Slim sized to fit in a purse or briefcase, or download to your favorite device.

"EASY Lifetime Diet & Exercise Guide" included inside in this book. This calorie counter and fitness guide provides the power for a lifetime of total success controlling your weight!

Written based on extensive research and input from nutritionists and fitness trainers. Includes important tips from people in their 20's, 30's, 40's, and 50's who have defied the odds and remained lean, toned, athletic, and healthy their entire lives. Read all of their secrets here! Read about what really works for lifetime weight control!

Easy Calorie Counter
& Fitness Guide

TABLE OF CONTENTS

Introduction

Welcome to the **Easy Calorie Counter & Fitness Guide**. Here is the power to control your weight forever. This is a guide to safe, simple, effective methods of managing weight, while promoting optimal health.

Nutrition experts agree, calories count first in weight management. This book is designed to help count calories accurately, quickly, and easily. Alphabetical listings make locating foods simple. To improve clarity and speed in locating food choices, the tables in this book are divided into 3 sections:

> **Beverages**
> **Foods**
> **Fast Food Restaurants**

Counting calories is a time-honored method for weight management. Nutrition experts agree that calories count first when trying to manage your weight. Other factors can then be addressed, including activity level, and how to balance the intake of carbohydrates, protein, fat, sodium, and other nutrients.

This book is designed to help make counting calories fast and easy. Precise and accurate alphabetical listings provide for quick calorie counts. Whether a pro or a novice at counting calories and nutrients, this book contains all the information needed. In the tables are all the foods people love to eat in the most common serving sizes. This includes the most popular foods, the most common foods, favorite fast food restaurants, brand names, beverages, and alcoholic beverages. There are about 3,500 listings in all.

To use this food counter, simply locate the choice of food or beverage in one of the three alphabetical sections:

Beverages
Foods
Fast Food Restaurants

Managing weight is so much easier with the right tools, including a good calorie counter, and a simple exercise plan. This calorie counter includes the EASY Lifetime Diet & Exercise Guide. Here, find all of the essential tools to manage weight, and shed those unwanted pounds and inches forever. This book is the power base for building a lifetime of good health, and the joy of achieving ideal body weight. The EASY Lifetime Diet & Exercise Guide also gives all the essential information needed to understand calories, healthy dieting, and exercise.

The formulas are included to calculate daily caloric requirements for achieving and maintaining ideal weight. Calorie expenditure is also covered, including how to burn calories faster. Also information about lifestyle activity factors, and how to increase activity levels to burn calories faster. Tips about safe and easy exercise, and plenty of diet tips and secrets. Calorie counting along with a simple exercise routine results in healthy weight management, with long-lasting results.

For the best results, read over the book, and especially, look at favorite foods, to get an idea of which foods are high in calories and which foods are low in calories. That will help make smart food choices every time you eat.

NOTES:

All listings are medium size or average portion size, unless specifically noted.

"Cooked" means the food is cooked without added fats, sauces, or sugars. This includes boiling, steaming, and heating in a microwave oven.

"Baked" and "Broiled" describe the normal methods of baking and broiling, using nonstick cooking spray, or minimal cooking oil. No other fats, sauces, or sugars added.

References for compiling this book include the United States Department of Agriculture (USDA) nutritional database, food manufacturers nutrient labels, and restaurants printed nutritional data. References for the diet and exercise data include the USDA database, WebMD, recommendations from nutritionists, exercise experts, and interviews with successful dieters age 20 to 60 years old.

The data is accurate at the time publication, however, food manufacturers may change their ingredients at any time without notice.

Abbreviation key

appx	approximately
as prep	prepared as instructed on package; the usual method
avg	average size
bev	beverage
cal	calorie
carb	carbohydrate
dia	diameter
fl oz	fluid ounce
g	gram(s)
"	inch(es)
Lb	pound
Lg	large
mcg	microgram(s)
med	medium
misc	miscellaneous
mg	milligram(s)
ml	milliliter(s)
oz	ounce
pc	piece
pkg	package
pkt	packet
prep	prepared
sm	small
svg	serving
sq	square
Tbsp	tablespoon
Tr	trace- less than 1 g or mg
tsp	teaspoon
w/	with
w/o	without

Metric Conversion Factors:

Volume	Multiply By	To Find Equivalent
Teaspoons	4.93	Milliliters
Tablespoons	14.79	Milliliters
Fluid ounces	29.57	Milliliters
Cups	0.24	Liters
Gallons	3.79	Liters

Weight	Multiply By	To Find Equivalent
Ounces	28.35	Grams
Pounds	0.45	Kilograms

Approximate Measure Equivalents:

Volume

1 Teaspoon = ...5 ml
1 Tablespoon =.....3 Teaspoons =............15 ml
2 Tablespoons =....1 fl oz = ...30 ml
4 Tablespoons =....¼ Cup = ...2 fl oz = ...59 ml
16 Tablespoons =...1 Cup = ...8 fl oz =.....237 ml
1 Cup =..........½ Pint =.......8 fl oz = ... 237 ml
2 Cups=.........1 Pint =.......16 fl oz = ...474 ml
2 Pints = ...1 Quart =....32 fl oz = ... 946 ml
1 Gallon = ...4 Quarts =..128 fl oz =   3.79 Liters

Weight

1 Ounce = 28 grams
1 Pound = 454 grams

BEVERAGES

BEVERAGE: (See Food and Fast Food Restaurants listed separately)	Serving Size	Calories
Amaretto, 53 proof	1.5 fl oz	175
Apple Juice	8 fl oz	115
Apple-Cranberry Juice	8 fl oz	115
Apple-Grape Juice	8 fl oz	130
Apple-Raspberry Juice	8 fl oz	120
Apricot Nectar	8 fl oz	140
BEER	...	...
Regular Beer	12 fl oz	150
Light Beer	12 fl oz	100
Dark beer	12 fl oz	160
Draft beer, regular	12 fl oz	150
Draft beer, light	12 fl oz	100
Dry beer	12 fl oz	130
Malt beer	12 fl oz	160
Bloody Mary	5 fl oz	150
Bourbon, 80 proof	1.5 fl oz	95
Brandy	...	...
80 proof	1.5 fl oz	95
Flavored, 60 proof, (Apricot Blackberry, or Cherry)	... 1.5 fl oz	... 180
Capri Sun juice drink	8 fl oz	122
Carbonated Beverages- see Soda	...	...
Carrot Juice	8 fl oz	95
Club Soda	12 fl oz	0
Cocoa / Chocolate Beverage, Hot	...	...
Regular, as prep	6 fl oz	170
Diet or sugarfree, as prep	6 fl oz	35
COFFEE	...	...
Brewed coffee, regular or decaf	6 fl oz	4
Instant coffee, regular or decaf	6 fl oz	4
Café Amaretto	6 fl oz	70
Café Latte	6 fl oz	115
Café Vienna	6 fl oz	70
Cappuccino	6 fl oz	65
Espresso	2 fl oz	5
French Vanilla Café	6 fl oz	70

BEVERAGE: (See Food and Fast Food Restaurants listed separately)	Serving Size	Calories
French Vanilla, sugarfree	6 fl oz	20
Hazelnut Belgian Cafe	6 fl oz	75
Swiss Mocha coffee	6 fl oz	75
Swiss Mocha coffee, sugarfree	6 fl oz	20
Viennese Chocolate coffee	6 fl oz	75
Coffee Cream – see Creamer	…	…
Coffee Liqueur, 53 proof	1.5 fl oz	175
Coke - see Soda	…	…
Cola - see Soda	…	…
Cranapple Drink	8 fl oz	170
Cranberry Juice Cocktail	8 fl oz	145
Cranberry-Grape Drink	8 fl oz	145
Creamer	…	…
Half & Half (cream & milk)	1 Tbsp	20
Half & Half (cream & milk)	1 cup	315
Liquid creamer Coffee-Mate	1 Tbsp	20
Powdered creamer Coffee-Mate	1 tsp	10
Crème de Menthe	1 fl oz	125
Crystal Light, all flavors	8 fl oz	5
Daiquiri, strawberry	4 fl oz	225
Diet Cola	12 fl oz	0
Diet or sugarfree Kool Aid	8 fl oz	5
Diet Soda	12 fl oz	0
Eggnog, plain	1 cup	345
Fruit Drink (5% to 10% juice)	…	…
All flavors	…	…
Regular	8 fl oz	135
Sugarfree	8 fl oz	5
Fruit Punch (10% Juice)	…	…
Regular	8 fl oz	130
Sugarfree	8 fl oz	5
Gatorade	8 fl oz	50
Gin, 80 proof	1.5 fl oz	95
Grape Juice	…	…
Canned or bottled, sweetened	8 fl oz	155
Frozen concentrate, sweetened,	…	…
as prep w/ water	8 fl oz	130
Unsweetened grape juice	8 fl oz	120
Grapefruit Juice	…	…
Fresh, squeezed, unsweetened	8 fl oz	95

BEVERAGE: (See Food and Fast Food Restaurants listed separately)	Serving Size	Calories
Fresh, squeezed, sugar	...	...
sweetened	8 fl oz	115
Fresh, squeezed, w/sugarfree	...	...
sweetener	8 fl oz	90
Canned, unsweetened	8 fl oz	95
Canned, sugar sweetened	8 fl oz	115
Frozen concentrate,	...	.
unsweetened, as prep w/ water	8 fl oz	100
Half & Half – see Creamer	...	...
Hawaiian Punch	...	...
Regular	8 fl oz	120
Sugarfree	8 fl oz	15
Hot Cocoa/Chocolate – see	...	...
Cocoa	...	...
Juice – see specific listings	...	...
Kool Aid	...	...
Sugar sweetened	8 fl oz	60
Sugarfree	8 fl oz	5
Unsweetened Packet	1 pkt	0
Lemon Juice	...	...
Fresh, squeezed, unsweetened	1 Tbsp	4
Canned or bottled, unsweetened	1 Tbsp	3
Canned or bottled, unsweetened	1 cup	50
Lemonade	...	...
Sugar Sweetened	8 fl oz	100
Sugarfree	8 fl oz	5
Lime Juice	...	...
Fresh or bottled, unsweetened	1 Tbsp	3
Fresh or bottled, unsweetened	1 cup	52
Limeade	...	...
Sugar sweetened	8 fl oz	100
Sugarfree	8 fl oz	5
Liqueur, 53 proof	...	...
Coffee or Fruit Flavored	1.5 fl oz	175
Mai Tai	5 fl oz	280
Margarita	5 fl oz	150
Martini	2.5 fl oz	155
MILK	...	...
White Milk	...	...
Whole milk, 3.3% fat	8 fl oz	150

BEVERAGE: (See Food and Fast Food Restaurants listed separately)	Serving Size	Calories
Reduced fat milk, 2% fat	8 fl oz	120
Lowfat milk, 1% fat	8 fl oz	102
Nonfat milk, (Skim milk)	8 fl oz	85
Nonfat instant,as prep w/water	8 fl oz	80
Nonfat instant,	…	…
dry powder only	1 cup	240
Chocolate Milk	…	…
Whole chocolate milk	8 fl oz	210
Reduced fat chocolate,2%	8 fl oz	180
Lowfat chocolate milk, 1%	8 fl oz	160
Misc Milk Products	…	…
Buttermilk	1 cup	100
Condensed, sweetened	1 cup	980
Evaporated whole milk	1 cup	340
Evaporated skim milk	1 cup	200
Malted milk, chocolate	1 cup	225
Malted milk, natural	1 cup	230
Soy milk	1 cup	81
Milk Shake – see Shake	…	…
Miso	1 cup	567
Nesquik, Chocolate, as prep	8 fl oz	210
Orange Juice	…	…
Fresh, squeezed, unsweetened	8 fl oz	112
Canned or bottled, unsweetened	8 fl oz	110
Frozen concentrate, as prep	8 fl oz	112
Peach Nectar	8 fl oz	135
Pear Nectar	8 fl oz	150
Pepsi – see Soda	…	…
Pina Colada	4.5 oz	260
Pineapple Grapefruit Juice	8 fl oz	120
Pineapple Juice	8 fl oz	140
Pineapple Orange Juice	8 fl oz	125
Prune Juice	8 fl oz	182
Root Beer	…	…
Regular	12 fl oz	170
Diet or sugarfree	12 fl oz	0
Rum, 80 proof	1.5 fl oz	95
Scotch, 80 proof	1.5 fl oz	95
Screwdriver	7 fl oz	160
Shake	…	…

BEVERAGE: (See Food and Fast Food Restaurants listed separately)	Serving Size	Calories
Regular milk shake	…	…
Chocolate	11 oz	360
Peach	11 oz	380
Strawberry	11 oz	395
Vanilla	11 0z	350
Low Carb shake	…	…
Atkins chocolate shake	11 oz	170
Atkins vanilla shake	11 oz	170
Soda / Cola / Soft Drink	…	...
(Carbonated Beverages)	…	…
Club Soda	12 fl oz	0
Cherry Cola, regular	12 fl oz	155
Cherry Cola, diet	12 fl oz	0
Coca Cola, Coke regular	12 fl oz	140
Coke, diet	12 fl oz	0
Cola	12 fl oz	150
Diet Cola	12 fl oz	0
Dr Pepper, regular	12 fl oz	150
Dr Pepper, diet	12 fl oz	0
Ginger Ale, regular	12 fl oz	125
Ginger Ale, diet	12 fl oz	0
Grape Soda, regular	12 fl oz	155
Grape Soda, diet	12 fl oz	0
Lemon Lime Soda, regular	12 fl oz	145
Lemon Lime Soda, diet	12 fl oz	0
Mountain Dew, regular	12 fl oz	170
Mountain Dew, diet	12 fl oz	0
Mr. Pibb, regular	12 fl oz	146
Mr. Pibb, diet	12 fl oz	0
Orange Soda, regular	12 fl oz	175
Orange Soda, diet	12 fl oz	0
Pepsi, regular	12 fl oz	150
Pepsi, diet	12 fl oz	0
RC Cola, regular	12 fl oz	160
RC Cola, diet	12 fl oz	0
Root Beer, Regular	12 fl oz	170
Root Beer, Diet	12 fl oz	0
Seven Up, regular	12 fl oz	150
Seven Up, diet	12 fl oz	0
Sprite, regular	12 fl oz	150
Sprite, diet	12 fl oz	0

BEVERAGE: (See Food and Fast Food Restaurants listed separately)	Serving Size	Calories
Tab	12 fl oz	1
Soft Drinks – see Soda	…	…
Sport Drink	12 fl oz	75
Sugarfree Beverage	…	.
(Also see specific listings)	…	.
Sugarfree Soda	12 fl oz	0
Sugarfree Kool Aid	8 fl oz	5
Sunny Delight, Citrus Punch	8 fl oz	125
Tang, regular	8 fl oz	115
Tang, sugarfree	8 fl oz	5
TEA, Hot or Iced	…	…
Regular, unsweetened	8 fl oz	2
Regular, sugar sweetened	8 fl oz	90
Regular, sugarfree sweetener	8 fl oz	4
Chamomile tea, unsweetened	8 fl oz	2
Chamomile tea, sugar sweetened	8 fl oz	90
Misc Types of Tea, Blends,	…	…
Black, Chinese, Orange Pekoe	…	…
Unsweetened	8 fl oz	2
Sugar sweetened	8 fl oz	90
Sugarfree sweetened	8 fl oz	4
Tequila	1.5 fl oz	100
Tequila Sunrise	5.5 fl oz	190
Tomato Juice	8 fl oz	41
V 8 Vegetable Juice, 1 Lg can	11 fl oz	70
Vegetable Juice	8 fl oz	46
Vodka	…	…
80 proof	1.5 oz	95
86 proof	1.5 oz	105
90 proof	1.5 oz	110
Water	8 fl oz	0
Whiskey	…	…
80 proof	1.5 oz	95
86 proof	1.5 oz	105
90 proof	1.5 oz	110
WINE	…	…
Dessert Wine, Dry	4 fl oz	150
Dessert Wine, Sweet	4 fl oz	180
Red Wine (table wine)	4 fl oz	85

BEVERAGE: (See Food and Fast Food Restaurants listed separately)	Serving Size	Calories
Rosè Wine	4 fl oz	85
White Wine (table wine)	4 fl oz	80
White Zinfandel	4 fl oz	85
Wine Cooler	5.5 oz	100
Wine Spritzer	5.5 oz	60

FOODS

FOOD: (See Beverages & Restaurants listed separately)	Serving Size	Calories
Accent Seasoning	¼ tsp	Tr
Alfalfa sprouts, fresh	1 cup	10
Almonds – see Nuts	...	...
Anchovy – see Fish	...	...
Anise Seed	1 Tbsp	28
Apple	...	...
Fresh, unpeeled, avg 2 ¾" dia	1	80
Fresh, peeled, sliced	1 cup	65
Dried	5 rings	80
Apple Butter	1 Tbsp	30
Apple Pie Filling	1 Tbsp	40
Applesauce	...	...
Sweetened	½ cup	97
Unsweetened	½ cup	52
Apricot	...	...
Fresh, medium size, 1.3 oz	1	17
Canned, in heavy syrup	1 cup	215
Canned, in juice	1 cup	115
Dried, halves	8 halves	80
Artichoke, Globe or French	...	...
Fresh, medium size, cooked	1	60
Fresh, cooked, drained	1 cup	84
Jerusalem artichoke, raw, sliced	1 cup	114
Arugula, raw	½ cup	3
Asparagus, cooked	...	...
Fresh, medium size spears	4 spears	14
Fresh, chopped pieces	1 cup	43
Frozen, spears	4 spears	17
Frozen, chopped pieces	1 cup	50
Canned, 5" spears	4 spears	14
Canned, chopped pieces	1 cup	46
Aspartame Sweetener	1 pkt	0
Avocado	...	...
California, 1/5 of whole	1 oz	50
Florida, 1/10 of whole	1 oz	30
Bacon – see Pork	...	...
Bacon Bits	1 Tbsp	31

FOOD: (See Beverages & Restaurants listed separately)	Serving Size	Calories
Bagel, 3 ½" dia	...	...
Plain	1	150
Cinnamon raisin	1	170
Egg	1	160
Multigrain	1	150
Baking Powder	1 tsp	2
Baking Soda	1 tsp	0
Bamboo Shoots, cooked	1 cup	25
Banana	...	...
Fresh, 7" long	1	110
Fresh, sliced	1 cup	140
Banana Split	1	510
Barley	...	...
Pearled, cooked	1 cup	195
Pearled, uncooked	1 cup	705
Basil, dried spice	½ tsp	3
Bean Sprouts (mung), cooked	1 cup	30
BEANS	...	...
Plain Beans, cooked w/o fats	...	...
Black beans	½ cup	115
Great Northern beans	½ cup	105
Green beans	½ cup	22
Kidney, Red beans	½ cup	112
Lima, large beans	½ cup	100
Lima, baby lima beans	½ cup	95
Pinto beans	½ cup	117
Soybeans	½ cup	135
Wax beans	½ cup	25
White beans	½ cup	150
Yellow beans	½ cup	22
Misc Bean Dishes, as prep	...	...
Baked beans,	...	...
plain or vegetarian	½ cup	118
Baked beans, BBQ style	½ cup	180
Baked beans w/frankfurters	½ cup	185
Baked beans w/tomato sauce	½ cup	125
Baked beans w/sweet sauce	½ cup	140
Beans w/ pork	½ cup	130
Black beans w/ rice	½ cup	150
Green bean casserole	½ cup	140
Green beans w/almonds	½ cup	60

FOOD: (See Beverages & Restaurants listed separately)	Serving Size	Calories
Red beans & rice	½ cup	130
Refried beans	½ cup	118
BEEF	...	...
Bottom Round, lean & fat	3 oz	235
lean only	3 oz	180
Brisket	3 oz	250
Chuck Blade, lean & fat	3 oz	295
lean only	3 oz	215
Corned Beef, canned	3 oz	215
Dried Beef, chipped	1 oz	45
Eye of Round, lean & fat	3 oz	195
lean only	3 oz	145
Flank Steak	3 oz	225
Ground Beef /	...	...
Hamburger meat, regular	3 oz	250
lean, 79%	3 oz	230
extra lean, 83%	3 oz	220
Liver of beef, fried	3 oz	185
Pastrami	2 oz	90
Porterhouse Steak	3.5 oz	325
Pot Roast, Chuck	3.5 oz	345
Prime Ribs	3.5 oz	400
Rib Roast, lean & fat	3 oz	305
lean only	3 oz	195
Roast Beef	3.5 oz	290
Short Ribs	3.5 oz	470
Sirloin Steak, lean & fat	3 oz	220
lean only	3 oz	165
T-bone Steak, lean & fat	3.5 oz	310
lean only	3.5 oz	250
Tenderloin Steak/ Top Loin	3.5 oz	305
Top Round	3.5 oz	215
(Weights for meat w/o bones,	...	...
as prep: braised, broiled,	...	...
grilled, simmered, or roasted. Also	...	...
see: Bologna, Hot Dog, Salami,	...	...
Sausage & specific entrées)	...	...
Beef & Macaroni	...	...
Healthy Choice, frozen	1 pkg	210
Beef Burgundy, Le Menu entrée	1 meal	315
Beef Jerky, ¾ oz	1	80

FOOD: (See Beverages & Restaurants listed separately)	Serving Size	Calories
Beef Meals – see Hamburger	…	…
Helper for ground beef meals	…	…
Beef Oriental, Lean Cuisine	1 meal	270
Beef Patties, Banquet entrée	1 meal	180
Beef Peppercorn, Lean Cuisine	1 meal	260
Beef Portabello, Lean Cuisine	1 meal	220
Beef Romanoff	1 cup	290
Beef Stew w/ Vegetables	1 cup	215
Beef Stroganoff, Stouffers entrée	1 meal	390
Beef Teriyaki w/ vegetables	1 cup	250
Beef Tips, Healthy Choice entrée	1 meal	260
Beef w/ Broccoli, Hunan style	1 cup	250
Beef w/Vegetables, Szechuan	1 cup	270
Beet Greens, chopped, cooked	½ cup	20
Beets	…	…
Fresh, cooked, slices	½ cup	38
Fresh, cooked, whole, 2" dia	1 whole	22
Canned, drained, slices	½ cup	27
Canned, drained, whole beet	1 whole	12
Biscuit, plain or buttermilk	…	…
Prep from recipe, 2 ½" dia	1	210
Prep from recipe, 4" dia	1	360
Refrigerated dough, baked	…	…
regular 2 ½" dia	1	95
reduced fat, 2 ¼" dia	1	65
Biscuit w/ Bacon	1	360
Biscuit w/ Egg & Sausage	1	540
Biscuit w/ Ham	1	330
Biscuit w/ Sausage	1	460
Blackberries	…	…
Fresh	1 cup	75
Frozen, no sugar added, thawed	1 cup	80
Blueberries	…	…
Fresh	1 cup	80
Frozen, sugar sweetened, thawed	1 cup	185
Bologna (thin 1/8" slices)	…	…
Beef or Pork, regular	2 slices	180
Beef or Pork, lowfat	2 slices	110
Beef or Pork, fat free	2 slices	60
Chicken or Turkey , regular	2 slices	160

FOOD: (See Beverages & Restaurants listed separately)	Serving Size	Calories
Chicken or Turkey, lowfat	2 slices	100
Chicken or Turkey, fat free	2 slices	60
Bouillon - see Soup	…	…
Bratwurst, Boars Head	1 wurst	300
Braunschweiger, 2 avg slices	2 oz	205
BREAD	…	…
(½" thick slice unless noted)	…	…
Banana bread, 1 ¼" slice	1 slice	195
Boston brown	1 slice	88
Bran'ola	1 slice	90
Bun, frankfurter, 1.4 oz, 5" long	1 bun	100
Bun, hamburger, 1.4 oz	1 bun	100
Bun, Lg, 7" long or 4" diameter	1 bun	200
Carb Style, Pepperidge Farms	1 slice	60
Carrot bread	1 slice	200
Cinnamon raisin bread	1 slice	90
Cornbread, 3" x 2"	1 piece	185
Cracked wheat bread	1 slice	65
Croissant, butter flavor, 4"	1	230
Egg bread, ¾" slice	1 slice	115
English muffin, regular	1 whole	135
English muffin, cinnamon/raisin	1 whole	140
French bread	1 slice	70
Garlic bread, ¾" thick	1 slice	150
Italian bread	1 slice	65
Multigrain bread	1 slice	65
Oat/Oatmeal bread	1 slice	73
Pita bread, 4" pita	1 whole	77
Pita bread, 6 ½" pita	1 whole	165
Potato bread	1 slice	100
Pumpernickel bread	1 slice	80
Raisin bread	1 slice	100
Reduced calorie bread	1 slice	45
Roll, cinnamon, w/glaze, 3" dia	1 roll	200
Roll, hard or kaiser	1 roll	170
Roll, soft, avg size, 1.4 oz	1 roll	100
Rye bread	1 slice	75
Sourdough bread	1 slice	70
Submarine bread, 7" long	1	200
Vienna bread	1 slice	70
Wheat bread	1 slice	65

FOOD: (See Beverages & Restaurants listed separately)	Serving Size	Calories
White bread	1 slice	65
White or Wheat, light bread	1 slice	45
(also see Bagel & Biscuit)	…	…
Bread Crumbs	…	…
Dry, grated	1 cup	430
Dry, seasoned, grated	1 cup	440
Soft crumbs	1 cup	120
Bread Stick	…	…
Crunchy w/sesame seeds, 0.4 oz	1	40
Soft, pizza flavored, 1.5 oz	1	130
Bread Stuffing – see Stuffing or	…	…
Bread Crumbs	…	…
Breakfast Sandwich, bacon, egg,	…	…
& cheese on English muffin	1 avg	370
(also see Biscuit sandwiches)	…	…
Broccoli	…	…
Fresh, raw, flowerets	3	9
Fresh, raw, spear, 5" long	1	9
Fresh, raw, chopped or diced	1 cup	25
Fresh, cooked, spear, 5" long	1	10
Fresh, chopped, cooked	1 cup	44
Frozen, flowerets & cuts, cooked	1 cup	52
Prep w/ butter sauce	½ cup	75
Broccoli & Rice Casserole	¾ cup	240
Broccoli Au gratin	½ cup	100
Broth - see Soup	…	…
Brownie, 2" square	…	…
With frosting	1	190
Without frosting	1	140
Fat Free	1	90
Brussels Sprouts	…	…
Fresh, cooked	1 cup	61
Frozen, cooked	1 cup	65
Prep w/ butter	½ cup	75
Bugles (snacks)	…	…
Regular	1 ¼ cup	150
Baked	1 ¼ cup	130
Nacho	1 ¼ cup	160
Ranch	1 ¼ cup	160
Sour cream & onion	1 ¼ cup	160
Bulgur	…	…

FOOD: (See Beverages & Restaurants listed separately)	Serving Size	Calories
Cooked	1 cup	150
Uncooked	1 cup	480
Bun - see Bread	...	...
Burrito	...	...
Bean & cheese	1	275
Bean & green chili	1	270
Beans & rice	1	200
Beef & bean	1	300
Beef & cheese	1	300
Chicken	1	260
Butter (also see margarine)	...	...
Regular stick, 4 sticks/pound	1 stick	815
Regular, salted or unsalted	1 Tbsp	100
Regular, salted or unsalted	1 tsp	34
Apple Butter	1 Tbsp	30
Cabbage	...	...
Green, raw, shredded	1 cup	18
Green, chopped, cooked	1 cup	33
Chinese cabbage (bok choy)	...	...
shredded, raw	1 cup	10
shredded, cooked	1 cup	20
Red cabbage, raw, shredded	1 cup	19
Savoy cabbage, raw, shredded	1 cup	19
Cabbage, Stuffed w/ beef or pork	1 avg	100
CAKE	...	...
(average slice of single layer	...	...
cake, 1/8 of 9", unless noted)	...	...
Angelfood cake, w/o frosting,	1 piece	125
Boston Cream Cake	1 piece	230
Carrot Cake, cream cheese icing	1 piece	485
Cheesecake, 1/6 of 17 oz cake	1 piece	260
Cheesecake w/chocolate	1 piece	580
Chocolate Cake	...	...
w/frosting	1 piece	390
w/o frosting	1 piece	290
Coffee Crumb Cake, 2.2 oz	1 piece	265
Cupcake – see Cupcakes	...	...
Devil's Food cake w/frosting	1 piece	395
Fat Free Cake,	...	...
w/o frosting	1 piece	80
w/sugar free glaze	1 piece	85

FOOD: (See Beverages & Restaurants listed separately)	Serving Size	Calories
Fruitcake, small slice	1 piece	160
Gingerbread	1 piece	265
Hummingbird	1 piece	595
Marble cake, w/o frosting	1 piece	255
Pineapple Upside Down Cake	1 piece	365
Pound Cake w/o glaze	1 piece	220
Shortcake, 3" dia	1 piece	225
Sponge Cake	1 piece	180
White Cake,	…	…
w/frosting	1 piece	395
w/o frosting	1 piece	265
Yellow Cake,	…	…
w/frosting	1 piece	390
w/o frosting	1 piece	260
CANDY & Chocolate Bars	…	…
Atomic FireBall, ¾" dia	1	24
Almond Joy, 1.7 oz bar	1 bar	240
Baby Ruth, 2.1 oz bar	1 bar	290
Bit-O-Honey, 2.1 oz	1 bar	185
BreathSavers, sugar free	1	5
Butterfinger, 2.1 oz bar	1 bar	280
Candy Cane, 0.5 oz	1 cane	55
Candy Corn	¼ cup	180
Caramel	…	…
regular caramel, 0.3 oz	1 piece	35
regular caramel, 2.5 oz	2.5 oz	270
chocolate caramel, 0.3 oz	1 piece	25
Carob	1 oz	155
Charms Blow Pop	1	60
Chewing Gum-see separately	…	…
Chocolate Bars	…	…
Hershey's Chocolate bar,	…	…
plain, 1.5 oz bar	1 bar	230
Hershey's Nugget, 10g	1 bar	52
Hershey's Snack Size, 17g	1 bar	90
with almonds, 1.45 oz	1 bar	220
with crispy rice, 1.55 oz	1 bar	230
with peanuts, 1.75 oz	1 bar	265
(see 'Chocolate for Baking'	…	…
listed separately)	…	…
Chocolate Coated Peanuts	10	205

FOOD: (See Beverages & Restaurants listed separately)	Serving Size	Calories
Chocolate Coated Raisins	10	40
Chocolate Kiss, Hershey's	4	102
Fifth Avenue bar, 2 oz	1 bar	195
Fruit Leather Bar	1 oz	95
Fruit Leather, small roll	1 roll	50
Fudge, chocolate, 0.6 oz piece	1 piece	65
Goobers, 1.4 oz	1	200
Gumdrops ¾" dia	5	64
Gummy Bears	10	85
Gummy Worms	10	285
Hard Candy, regular, 1" dia	…	…
Butterscotch or Coffee flavor	2	42
Cinnamon, Fruit, Mint flavor	2	40
Hard Candy, sugar free	…	…
Baskin Robbins, sugarfree	…	…
Fruit or Chocolate Mint	2	20
Brachs, sugar free Cinnamon	3	35
Life Savers, sugar free	4	30
Sweet 'N Low Fruit Flavors	5	30
Sweet 'N Low Butterscotch	5	30
Sweet 'N Low Coffee	5	30
Jawbreaker, regular size, ¾" dia	1	24
Jawbreaker, large size, 1" dia	1	40
Jelly Beans, regular size	10	100
Jelly Beans, small pieces	10	40
Kit Kat bar, 1.5 oz	1 bar	215
Krackel bar, 1.5 oz	1 bar	220
Licorice, 1.4 oz pkg	1.4 oz	135
LifeSavers	2	20
Lollipop, Charms Blow Pop 15g	1	60
Lollipop, large, 14 g	1	50
Lollipop, small, Dum Dum, 5 g	1	24
M&M candy, plain	10	34
M&M candy, w/ nuts	10	103
Mars Almond bar, 1.75 oz	1 bar	235
Marshmallow, avg size	1	23
Milky Way, reg size, 2.15 oz	1 bar	258
Milky Way, small, fun size	1 bar	76
Mints, pastel, ½" square	10	75
Mounds, 1.9 oz bar	1 bar	255
Mr. Goodbar, 1.75 oz	1 bar	265

FOOD: (See Beverages & Restaurants listed separately)	Serving Size	Calories
Oh Henry, 2 oz bar	1 bar	245
Nestle Crunch bar, 1.55 oz	1 bar	230
Peanut Brittle	1 oz	130
Peppermint Pattie, 1.5 oz	1 pattie	165
Raisinets, 1.6 oz pkg	1 pkg	185
Reese's Peanut Butter Cups	…	…
regular size cups	2 cups	245
miniature size cups	2 cups	42
Reese's Pieces, 1.6 oz pkg	1 pkg	225
Reese Sticks, 0.6 oz bar	1 bar	90
Rolo caramels	9 piece	220
Skittles, 2.3 oz pkg	1 pkg	265
Skor toffee bar, 1.4 oz	1 bar	220
Snickers bar, regular size, 2 oz	1 bar	275
Snickers bar, small fun size	1 bar	72
Special Dark, miniature bar	1 bar	46
Starburst Fruit Chews, 2 oz pkg	1 pkg	235
Starlight Mints, 1" dia	3	56
Sucker – see Lollipop	…	…
Three Musketeers, 2.1 oz bar	1 bar	250
Toffee, 1.4 oz bar	1 bar	220
Tootsie Roll, 1 oz	1 oz	110
Twizzlers, Cherry, 2.5 oz pkg	1 pkg	135
Cannelloni, Cheese	…	…
Lean Cuisine entrée	1 meal	250
Cantaloupe	…	…
Fresh, medium size, 5" dia	½	98
Fresh, wedge 1/8 melon	1 wedge	25
Fresh, cubed	1 cup	55
Carambola (starfruit)	…	…
Fresh, 3 ½", whole	1	30
Fresh, sliced	1 cup	36
Caramels – see candy	…	…
Carrot	…	…
Fresh, raw, whole, 7 ½" long	1	32
Fresh, raw, shredded	1 cup	47
Fresh, baby carrots	2	12
Fresh, cooked, slices	1 cup	65
Frozen, cooked, slices	1 cup	69
Canned, drained, slices, cooked	1 cup	57
Glazed carrots	¾ cup	280

FOOD: (See Beverages & Restaurants listed separately)	Serving Size	Calories
Cashew – see Nuts	…	…
Casserole, see specific listings	…	…
Catsup, regular	1 Tbsp	18
Restaurant size packet	1 pkt	10
Cauliflower	…	…
Fresh, raw, flowerets	3	9
Fresh, raw, chopped or diced	1 cup	25
Fresh, flowerets, cooked	3	12
Fresh, chopped, cooked	1 cup	30
Frozen, cuts, cooked	1 cup	35
Prep w/ butter	¾ cup	100
Prep w/ cheese sauce	¾ cup	110
Cavatelli	1 cup	400
Caviar – see Fish	…	…
Cayenne, dried spice	¼ tsp	1
Caesar Salad	4 oz	200
Celery	…	…
Fresh, raw, stalk, 7 ½" long	1 stalk	6
Fresh, raw, diced	1 cup	19
Cooked, stalk 7 ½" long	1 stalk	6
Cooked, diced pieces	1 cup	27
Celery Seed	1 tsp	8
CEREAL	…	…
All-Bran	½ cup	80
Apple Jacks	1 cup	116
Cap'n Crunch, regular	¾ cup	107
Crunchberries	¾ cup	104
Peanut Butter Crunchy	¾ cup	112
Cheerios Cereal, regular	1 cup	110
Apple Cinnamon Cheerios	¾ cup	118
Chex Cereal, Corn	1 cup	113
Honey Nut	¾ cup	117
Multi Bran	1 cup	170
Rice	1¼ cup	117
Wheat	1 cup	104
Cinnamon Toast Crunch	¾ cup	124
Cocoa Krispies	¾ cup	120
Cocoa Puffs	1 cup	120
Corn Flakes	1 cup	105
Corn Pops	1 cup	118
Cream of Wheat, as prep	1 cup	130

FOOD: (See Beverages & Restaurants listed separately)	Serving Size	Calories
Crispix	1 cup	108
Fruit Loops	1 cup	117
Frosted Flakes	1 cup	120
Frosted Mini Wheats	…	…
regular size	1 cup	175
bite size	1 cup	190
Golden Grahams	¾ cup	116
Granola Cereal, Nature Valley	¾ cup	250
Honey Nut Cheerios	1 cup	115
Kix Cereal, regular	1¼ cup	114
Kix Berry Berry	¾ cup	120
Life Cereal, regular	¾ cup	120
Life Cinnamon Cereal	1 cup	190
Lucky Charms	1 cup	116
Malt O Meal, as prep	1 cup	122
Oat Cereal, Cheerios type	1 cup	110
Oatmeal, warm - see Oatmeal	…	…
Peanut Butter Puffed Cereal	¾ cup	130
Product 19	1 cup	110
Puffed Rice Cereal	1 cup	56
Puffed Wheat Cereal	1 cup	44
Raisin Bran Cereal	1 cup	180
Raisin Nut Bran	1 cup	210
Rice Crispies	1 ¼ cup	124
Shredded wheat cereal,	…	…
frosted biscuits	1 cup	190
Smacks Cereal	¾ cup	105
Special K	1 cup	115
Total	¾ cup	105
Trix Cereal	1 cup	122
Wheat Bran Flakes	¾ cup	95
Wheaties	1 cup	110
Cereal Bar	…	…
Granola Chocolate Chip-small	1 bar	90
Plain- regular size bar	1 bar	135
Fruit filled- regular size bar	1 bar	145
Chalupa	…	…
Beef	1	380
Chicken	1	360
Nacho cheese & beef	1	370
Nacho cheese & chicken	1	350

FOOD: (See Beverages & Restaurants listed separately)	Serving Size	Calories
Nacho cheese & steak	1	350
CHEESE	...	...
American, pasteurized cheese	...	...
regular	1 oz	105
fat free	1 slice	25
Blue cheese	1 oz	100
Camembert 1.3 oz	1 pc	114
Cheddar cheese	...	...
regular, 1 ounce slice	1 slice	115
1 inch cube	1 slice	68
shredded	1 cup	455
lowfat	1 oz	50
fat free	1 slice	25
Cheese food, pasteurized	1 oz	93
Cheese spread, pasteurized	1 oz	82
Colby cheese	1 oz	112
Cottage cheese	...	...
regular, creamed, 4% fat	...	...
large curd	1 cup	233
small curd	1 cup	217
with fruit	1 cup	279
lowfat, 2% fat	1 cup	203
lowfat, 1% fat	1 cup	164
fat free	1 cup	160
dry curd, uncreamed, 0.5% fat	1 cup	123
Cream cheese	...	...
regular cream	1 oz	100
regular cream	1 Tbsp	50
lowfat/light	1 Tbsp	35
fat free	1 Tbsp	15
Feta cheese	1 oz	75
Fontina cheese	1 oz	110
Goat cheese, soft	1 oz	75
Jalapeno jack cheese	1 oz	90
Monterey jack cheese	1 oz	105
Mozzarella cheese	...	...
regular, 1 ounce slice	1 slice	80
shredded, 2 oz	½ cup	160
fat free	1 slice	25
Muenster cheese, sliced	1 oz	105
Neufchatel cheese	1 oz	75

FOOD: (See Beverages & Restaurants listed separately)	Serving Size	Calories
Parmesan cheese	...	...
grated, 1 cup	1 cup	455
grated, 1 tablespoon	1 Tbsp	25
Provolone cheese	1 oz	100
Ricotta cheese	...	...
regular	1 cup	430
part skim	1 cup	340
fat free	1 cup	240
Romano cheese, grated	1 oz	110
Roquefort, sheep's milk	1 oz	105
Swiss cheese	...	...
regular, 1 ounce slice	1 slice	105
fat free	1 slice	25
Cheeseburger (see hamburger)	...	...
Cheese Puffs (about 25)	1 oz	160
Cheese Puffs Balls (2 ½ cups)	1 oz	160
Cheese Spread	...	...
Cheez Whiz	2 Tbsp	90
Velveeta	2 Tbsp	80
Cheetos (snacks)	...	...
Curls (about 15)	1 oz	150
Puffs (about 25)	1 oz	160
Cherries	...	...
Fresh, sweet	10	50
Sour, canned, water pack	1 cup	90
Cherry Pie Filling, canned	3 oz	80
Chestnut – see Nuts	...	...
Chewing Gum,	...	...
Stick Gum, 2 ¾" long	...	...
Regular stick gum	1 stick	10
Wrigley's Extra, sugarfree	1 stick	5
Carefree, sugarfree	1 stick	5
Bubble Yum, all regular flavors	1	25
Dentyne Ice, all flavors	2	5
Gum Balls, small, ½" dia balls	5	40
Gum Balls, Lg, 1 ¼" dia balls	1	32
Grapermelon, Wrigley's, ¾"	2	10
Strappleberry, Wrigley's, ¾"	2	10
Trident, all flavors, 1" sticks	1 stick	5
Chex Mix, 1 oz	2/3 cup	120
CHICKEN	...	...

FOOD: (See Beverages & Restaurants listed separately)	Serving Size	Calories
Giblets, simmered, chopped	1 cup	230
Fried Chicken, batter dipped	…	…
½ Breast, about 4 oz	½	365
Drumstick, avg size	1	195
Thigh, avg size	1	240
Wing, avg size	2	160
Strips, dark meat	3 oz	205
Strips, white meat	3 oz	175
Liver of chicken, simmered	1	31
Neck, simmered	1	32
Roasted or Broiled Chicken	…	…
½ Breast, about 3.5 oz meat	½	165
Drumstick, avg size	1	75
Thigh, avg size	1	110
White meat w/ skin	3.5 oz	280
White meat, skinless	3.5 oz	170
Dark meat w/ skin	3.5 oz	320
Dark meat skinless	3.5 oz	190
Canned, boneless	5 oz	235
Stewed Chicken	…	…
Light & dark meat, diced	1 cup	330
Wings, Buffalo, hot	4	220
Wings, skinless, unbreaded	4	220
(Other Chicken Products, see:	…	…
Bologna, Hot Dog, Salami,	…	…
Sausage & specific entrées)	…	…
Chicken a la King	1 cup	320
Chicken Alfredo	1 cup	300
Chicken & Broccoli Alfredo	1 ½ cup	300
Chicken Cacciatoré	…	…
Healthy Choice entrée	1 meal	250
Lean Cuisine entrée	1 meal	280
Chicken Cordon Blue	…	…
Le Menu entrée	1 meal	460
Chicken Dijon, Healthy Choice	1 meal	270
Chicken Francesca	…	…
Healthy Choice entrée	1 meal	330
Chicken Kiev, Tyson entrée	1 meal	440
Chicken Marsala, Tyson entrée	1 meal	180
Chicken Nuggets	…	…
Banquet entrée	1 meal	410

FOOD: (See Beverages & Restaurants listed separately)	Serving Size	Calories
Morton entrée	1 meal	320
Chicken Parmagiana	…	…
Banquet entrée	1 meal	290
Healthy Choice entrée	1 meal	300
Le Menu entrée	1 meal	395
Chicken Roll, light meat	2 oz	90
Chicken Teriyaki w/vegetables	1 cup	200
Chicken w/Sweet & Sour Sauce	1 cup	320
Chicken w/Vegetables	…	…
Lean Cuisine entrée	1 meal	250
Chickpeas, cooked	½ cup	140
Chili Powder	1 tsp	8
Chili w/Beans	1 cup	270
Chili Con Carne w/Beans	1 cup	255
Chimichanga	…	…
Beans & cheese	1	300
Beef & cheese	1	425
Chicken & cheese	1	350
Chips – see Corn Chips, Potato Chips & other specific listings	…	…
Chives, raw, chopped	1 Tbsp	1
Chocolate for Baking (Also see 'Candy' for other chocolates)	…	…
Chocolate Chips, milk, regular	1 cup	860
Chocolate Chips, semisweet	1 cup	805
Chocolate Chips, white	1 cup	915
Unsweetened for baking, solid	1 sq	148
Unsweetened, liquid	1 oz	134
Chow Mein	…	…
Beef chow mein	1 ½ cup	170
Chicken chow mein	1 ½ cup	160
Cilantro, raw	1 tsp	Tr
Cinnamon	1 tsp	6
Cinnamon Sweet Roll	…	…
With glaze, 3" dia	1	200
With raisins & glaze, 3" dia	1	225
With raisins & glaze, 4 ½" dia	1	510
Clam Chowder - see Soup	…	…
Clams – see Fish/Seafood	…	…
Cloves, ground	1 tsp	6

FOOD: (See Beverages & Restaurants listed separately)	Serving Size	Calories
Cocoa, unsweetened powder	1 Tbsp	15
Cocoa, unsweetened, powder	1 cup	240
Coconut	…	…
Fresh piece, 2" x 2" x ½"	1 piece	160
Fresh, shredded, not packed	1 cup	285
Dried, sweetened, flaked	1 cup	465
Coleslaw	½ cup	62
Collards	…	…
Fresh, chopped, cooked	1 cup	49
Frozen, chopped, cooked	1 cup	61
Condiments, see Sauce,	…	…
or see specific listing	…	…
COOKIES 2 ¼" diameter	…	…
unless noted	…	…
Animal Crackers, 1" dia	8	60
Butter Cookie	1	50
Chocolate Chip, regular	1	80
Chocolate Chip, reduced fat	1	70
Chocolate Chip, sugar free	1	70
Coconut cookie	1	75
Fig Newton	2	110
Molasses cookie	1	80
Oatmeal w/ raisins	1	75
Oatmeal, plain	1	70
Oatmeal, sugarfree	1	70
Peanut Butter, plain	1	80
Peanut Butter w/ nuts	1	90
Pecan Shortbread cookie	1	75
Sandwich cookie, w/ filling,	…	…
1 ½" dia, round,	…	…
chocolate w/ creme filling	1	50
sugar w/ peanut butter filling	1	60
vanilla w/ creme filling	1	50
Shortbread cookie, plain	1	45
Shortbread w/fudge stripes	1	65
Sugar Cookie, regular	1	65
Sugar Cookie, reduced fat	1	55
Wafer, creme filled,	…	…
2 ½" x 1" rectangles,	…	…
chocolate, creme filling	3	140
sugarfree, w/ filling	3	100

FOOD: (See Beverages & Restaurants listed separately)	Serving Size	Calories
vanilla, creme filling	3	130
Wafer, Vanilla, round, 1 ½" dia	4	75
Cooking Spray, nonstick	…	…
¼ second spray	1 spray	0
Corn	…	…
Sweet White, 5" cob, cooked	1 ear	83
Sweet Yellow, on 5" cob,	…	…
fresh, cooked, 5" cob	1 ear	83
frozen, cooked, 5" cob	1 ear	75
frozen, cooked, kernels	½ cup	65
canned, kernels, vacuum pack	½ cup	83
canned, cream style kernels	½ cup	92
Prep w/butter & herb sauce	¾ cup	180
Corn Cake, butter flavor	1	40
(also see Rice Cake)	…	…
Corn Chips	…	…
Regular	1 oz	160
Barbecue flavor	1 oz	170
Ranch flavor	1 oz	150
Reduced fat	1 oz	130
Tortilla type	1 oz	140
Doritos corn chips	12 pc	140
Doritos nacho cheese	12 pc	140
Doritos ranch	12 pc	140
Doritos spicy nacho	12 pc	135
Fritos corn chips, regular	28 pc	160
Fritos BBQ corn chips	28 pc	160
Fritos Chili cheese corn chips	28 pc	160
Tostitos corn chips, round	13 pc	150
Tostitos baked	13 pc	110
Tostitos nacho	6 pc	150
Tostitos restaurant style	7 pc	140
Corn Grits (hominy) – see Grits	…	…
Corn Syrup	1 Tbsp	56
Cornbread, 3" x 2"	1 piece	185
Corned Beef, canned	3 oz	215
Corned Beef Hash	1 cup	440
Cornish Hen, roasted	4 oz	200
Cornmeal, yellow, dry form	…	…
Whole grain	1 cup	440
Self rising	1 cup	490

FOOD: (See Beverages & Restaurants listed separately)	Serving Size	Calories
Cornstarch	1 Tbsp	30
Cottage cheese – see Cheese	…	…
Crabcake	1	150
Cracker Jacks	½ cup	120
CRACKERS	…	…
Butter flavor, round, 2" dia	5	80
Cheese crackers, 1" squares	10	50
Chicken in a Biskit	12	160
Club crackers	4	70
Club crackers, Keebler Club	4	50
Graham crackers, 2 ½" sq	3	90
Matzo, plain, 6" square	1	120
Melba toast, plain	4	80
Oat Thins	9	70
Oyster crackers	25	65
Ritz Bitz w/peanut butter	13	150
Ritz crackers, regular	5	80
Ritz crackers, reduced fat	5	70
Saltine crackers	4	50
Sandwich crackers, 1 ½" dia,	…	…
cheese crackers	2	65
peanut butter crackers	2	65
Snack crackers, round, 2" dia	5	80
Sociables	7	80
Town House crackers	5	80
Triscuit wafers	7	140
Vegetable crackers, thin squares	7	80
Wheat Thins	9	60
Wheatables	8	70
Whole wheat, thin squares	8	75
Zwieback	2	70
Cranberries	…	.
Fresh, raw, unsweetened	½ cup	23
Dried, sweetened	¼ cup	90
Cranberry Relish	¾ cup	330
Cranberry relish w/walnuts	¾ cup	365
Cranberry Sauce, sweet, canned	1 slice	85
Cream Cheese - see Cheese	…	…
Cream of Tartar	1 tsp	8
Cream of Wheat Cereal, as prep	1 cup	130
Cream, Whipped Topping	…	…

FOOD: (See Beverages & Restaurants listed separately)	Serving Size	Calories
Light	1 cup	700
Light	1 Tbsp	45
Heavy	1 cup	820
Heavy	1 Tbsp	50
Pressurized in can	1 Tbsp	8
Creamer-see Beverages, Creamer	…	…
Croissant, butter flavor, 4"	1	230
Croissant w/Egg, Bacon, Cheese	1	415
Croissant w/Sausage	1	440
Croutons, seasoned	½ cup	92
Cucumber	…	…
Fresh, peeled, whole, 8" long	1	35
Fresh, peeled, sliced	1 cup	14
Fresh, unpeeled, whole 8" long	1	40
Fresh, unpeeled, sliced	1 cup	14
Cucumber Salad, mayo dressing	¾ cup	120
Cupcake, w/frosting, avg size, 2 ¾" dia x 2 ¼" tall	… …	… …
Banana	1	190
Blueberry	1	185
Chocolate	1	195
Chocolate w/ crème filling	1	190
Coconut w/ crème filling	1	200
Strawberry	1	185
Vanilla	1	190
Curry Powder	1 tsp	7
Custard	½ cup	170
Dandelion Greens, cooked	1 cup	35
Danish Pastry	…	…
Cheese, 4" dia	1	265
Cinnamon & raisin, 4" dia	1	260
Fruit filled, 4" dia	1	260
Large, Cheese w/ fruit, 5" x 3"	1	425
Dates, pitted	…	…
Whole	5 dates	115
Chopped	1 cup	490
Dessert – see Ice Cream, Frozen Dessert, or specific listing	… …	… …
Dessert Filling - see specific listing	… …	… …

FOOD: (See Beverages & Restaurants listed separately)	Serving Size	Calories
Dessert Topping – see Topping	...	...
Dill Weed, raw, sprigs	5	Tr
Dip	...	...
Avocado	1 Tbsp	30
Bacon	1 Tbsp	30
French Onion	1 Tbsp	25
Ranch	1 Tbsp	30
Sour Cream & Chives, regular	1 Tbsp	30
Sour Cream & Chives, light	1 Tbsp	15
Doughnut	...	...
Cake Doughnuts	...	...
Regular ring type, 3" dia	...	...
Plain	1	200
Powdered sugar	1	240
Chocolate frosting	1	270
Vanilla frosting & sprinkles	1	280
Holes or Munchkins	...	...
Cinnamon coated	4	250
Plain	4	220
Powdered sugar	4	250
Cruller glazed & frosted	...	...
w/chocolate	1	280
Yeast Doughnuts	...	...
Regular ring type, 3" dia	...	...
Glazed	1	200
Glazed & frosted w/vanilla	1	250
Glazed & frosted	...	...
w/chocolate & sprinkles	1	270
Holes or Munchkins	...	...
Glazed	5	200
Sugar coated	6	220
Filled doughnuts	...	...
Vanilla iced, crème filled	1	360
Powdered & strawberry	...	...
filled	1	260
Dressing – see Salad Dressing	...	...
Dried Fruit – see specific listings, and Trail Mix	... ...	... ...
Duck, roasted, ½ Duck, meat only	½ duck	445
Dumpling, steamed, filled w/meat, poultry, or seafood	... 2	... 85

FOOD: (See Beverages & Restaurants listed separately)	Serving Size	Calories
Pot sticker dumpling	2	144
Éclair, 5" x 2"	1	260
EGGs	...	...
Raw Eggs	...	...
1 medium whole egg	1	65
1 large whole egg	1	75
1 extra large whole egg	1	85
1 yolk only, large	1	60
1 white only, large	1	15
Prepared Eggs (1 Lg egg/svg)	...	...
deviled	1	120
hard boiled, whole	1	75
hard boiled, chopped	1 cup	210
omelet, plain, milk added	1	105
pan fried in margarine	1	92
poached	1	75
scrambled w/margarine & milk	... 1	... 100
Egg Substitute or imitation	¼ cup	35
Eggplant	...	...
Cubed, cooked	1 cup	28
Fried sticks	½ cup	240
Eggplant Parmagiana	½ cup	265
Eggroll	...	...
Chicken, Chun King entrée	1 meal	170
Chicken, La Choy entrée	1 meal	170
Pork, Chun King entrée	1 meal	170
Pork eggroll, 4" long, 1 avg	1	165
Shrimp, Chun King entrée	1 meal	150
Enchilada	...	...
Beef, Banquet entrée	1meal	380
Beef, Patio entrée	1 meal	350
Cheese, Banquet entrée	1 meal	340
Chicken, Banquet entrée	1 meal	360
Enchirito	...	...
Beef	1	370
Chicken	1	350
Steak	1	350
Endive, raw, chopped	1 cup	9
Energy Bar, low carb	...	...
Atkins Advantage Chocolate	1 bar	220

FOOD: (See Beverages & Restaurants listed separately)	Serving Size	Calories
Atkins Advantage S'mores	1 bar	220
English Muffin	...	...
Regular	1 whole	135
Cinnamon raisin	1 whole	140
English Muffin w/Egg, Cheese, & Canadian Bacon	... 1	... 290
Equal sweetener	1 pkt	0
Fajita, Chicken, Healthy Choice	1 meal	260
Fettuccini Alfredo, w/ beef	1 cup	310
Fig, fresh or dried, large	2	98
FISH / SEAFOOD	...	...
Abalone, fried	3 oz	160
Anchovy, canned in oil	5	42
Bass	...	...
black, baked	3 oz	260
striped, baked	3 oz	105
Bluefish, baked	3 oz	135
Catfish	...	...
baked or broiled	3 oz	130
breaded, fried	3 oz	195
Caviar, black or red	2 Tbsp	80
Clams	...	...
breaded, fried	¾ cup	450
canned, drained	3 oz	125
canned, drained	1 cup	235
raw	3 oz	63
raw	1 med	11
steamed	3 oz	125
Cod, baked or broiled	3 oz	90
Crab, Alaska king	...	...
steamed	3 oz	82
steamed	1 leg	130
Crab, blue	...	...
steamed	3 oz	88
canned	1 cup	135
Crab, imitation crab meat	3 oz	88
Crab cake, w/egg, fried	1 cake	95
Dolphinfish filet	4 oz	115
Fish fillet, breaded, fried	3 oz	190
Fish stick, breaded, fried, 3 x 1"	2 sticks	76
Flounder	...	...

FOOD: (See Beverages & Restaurants listed separately)	Serving Size	Calories
baked or broiled	3 oz	100
breaded, fried fillet	3 oz	190
Grouper, baked or broiled	3 oz	100
Haddock	...	...
baked or broiled	3 oz	95
breaded, fried fillet	3 oz	195
Halibut	...	...
baked or broiled	3 oz	120
breaded, fried fillet	3 oz	210
Herring, pickled	3 oz	225
Lobster, steamed	3 oz	85
Lobster, imitation meat	3 oz	90
Mackerel	...	...
baked or broiled	3 oz	225
mackerel, jack, canned	1 cup	295
Mahi Mahi filet	4 oz	115
Monkfish, baked or broiled	3 oz	130
Mussels, steamed	3 oz	145
Orange roughy, baked or broiled	3 oz	75
Oyster	...	...
raw meat	1 cup	170
raw meat	6 med	55
breaded, fried	3 oz	165
Perch, baked or broiled	3 oz	105
Pike, baked or broiled	3 oz	95
Pollock, baked or broiled	3 oz	95
Pompano, baked or broiled	3 oz	180
Rockfish, baked or broiled	3 oz	105
Salmon	...	...
baked or broiled	3 oz	185
canned, pink	3 oz	118
smoked, chinook	3 oz	100
Sardine, canned in oil, drained	3 oz	175
Scallop	...	...
breaded, fried	6 large	200
steamed	3 oz	95
Shark	...	...
Pacific shark, baked	3 oz	130
thrasher, baked	3 oz	85
Shrimp	...	...
breaded, fried	2 large	110

FOOD: (See Beverages & Restaurants listed separately)	Serving Size	Calories
breaded, fried	3 oz	205
canned, drained	3 oz	100
Snapper, baked or broiled	3 oz	110
Sole	…	…
baked or broiled	3 oz	100
breaded, fried fillet	3 oz	190
Squid, fried	3 oz	150
Swordfish	…	…
baked	3 oz	130
broiled	4 oz	170
Trout, baked or broiled	3 oz	145
Tuna	…	…
baked or broiled	3 oz	120
canned in oil, drained	3 oz	170
canned in water, chunk light	3 oz	100
canned in water, solid white	3 oz	110
tuna salad, oil packed, w/mayo	½ cup	190
tuna salad, water packed, w/	…	…
light mayo type dressing	½ cup	130
Whiting, baked or broiled	3 oz	100
Fish & Chips, Swanson entrée	1 meal	495
Fish & Macaroni w/cheese Stouffers entrée	… 1 meal	… 460
Fish Baked w/Lemon Pepper Healthy Choice entrée	… 1 meal	… 290
Fish Florentine, Lean Cuisine	1 meal	240
Fish Sandwich, 3 oz fried fish fillet with tarter sauce & cheese	… 1 avg	… 530
Flank Steak – see Beef	…	…
Flour, unsifted	…	…
All purpose flour, white	1 cup	455
Bread flour	1 cup	495
Buckwheat flour, whole groat	1 cup	400
Cake or pastry flour	1 cup	495
Carob flour	1 cup	230
Self-rising flour, white	1 cup	443
Whole wheat flour	1 cup	407
Frankfurter – see Hot Dog	…	…
Freezer Pop – see Frozen Dessert	…	…
French Fries Frozen, heated,	… …	… …

FOOD: (See Beverages & Restaurants listed separately)	Serving Size	Calories
thin, shoestring strips, 3 oz	20 fries	130
thick or crinkle cuts, 4.5 oz	20 fries	195
Restaurant type, regular fries	1 med	350
Curly Cheddar Fries	1 med	460
Curly Fries	1 med	400
French Toast	2 slices	250
Fried Chicken – see Chicken	…	…
Fried Rice – see Rice	…	…
Frijoles	1 cup	225
Frosting	…	…
Chocolate	1 Tbsp	75
Vanilla	1 Tbsp	80
Frozen Dessert	…	…
(also see Ice Cream)	…	…
Freezer Pop – (long tubes)_	…	…
Regular, fruit flavored, 1.5 oz	1	25
Sugar free, fruit flav, 1.5 oz	2	4
Frozen chocolate log cake	1 slice	280
Frozen chocolate round cake	1 slice	340
Fruit & Juice Bar, 2.5 oz	1	65
Fudge Bar, 1.75 oz	1	65
Ice Pop Bar, 2 oz	1	45
Italian Ices	½ cup	65
Popsicle, 4 oz	1	90
Vanilla Sandwich bar	1	220
Fruit (see specific listings)	…	…
Mixed, canned, w/light syrup	1 cup	150
Mixed, frozen, sweetened	1 cup	245
Fruit Cocktail	…	…
Canned in heavy syrup	1 cup	180
Canned in juice	1 cup	110
Fruit Salad, mixed diced fruits	¾ cup	70
Fudge	…	…
Chocolate fudge, plain	1 oz	110
Chocolate fudge w/ nuts	1 oz	125
Vanilla fudge, plain	1 oz	105
Vanilla fudge, w/nuts	1 oz	120
Funyuns (snacks)	13	140
Garlic, raw	1 clove	4
Garlic Powder or Salt	1 tsp	8

FOOD: (See Beverages & Restaurants listed separately)	Serving Size	Calories
Gelatin (Jello)	…	…
Banana, regular	½ cup	80
Banana, sugar free	½ cup	10
Cherry, regular	½ cup	75
Cherry, sugar free	½ cup	10
Orange, regular	½ cup	75
Orange, sugar free	½ cup	10
Raspberry, regular	½ cup	75
Raspberry, sugar free	½ cup	10
Strawberry , regular	½ cup	75
Strawberry, sugar free	½ cup	10
Gordita	…	…
Beef & cheese	1	310
Chicken & cheese	1	290
Steak & cheese	1	290
Granola Bar	…	…
Low fat, fruit variety,small bar	1 bar	90
Plain granola bar	1 bar	135
Chocolate chip	1 bar	150
Chocolate chip & peanuts	1 bar	160
Coconut	1 bar	140
Raisin	1 bar	140
Grapefruit, pink, red, or white	…	…
fresh, 3 ¾" dia	1	80
canned, in juice	1 cup	115
canned, in light syrup	1 cup	150
Grapes, seeded	…	…
Fresh, medium size, all types	10	35
Fresh, small or medium size	1 cup	115
Gravy	…	…
Beef	¼ cup	40
Chicken	¼ cup	32
Country Sausage	¼ cup	60
Mushroom	¼ cup	30
Pork	¼ cup	38
Turkey	¼ cup	31
Grits, corn (hominy), as prep	1 cup	145
Ground Beef – see Beef	…	…
Guava, raw, med size	1	45
Gum – see Chewing Gum	…	…
HAM (also see Pork)	…	…

FOOD: (See Beverages & Restaurants listed separately)	Serving Size	Calories
Canned, regular, roasted	3 oz	155
lean, roasted	3 oz	130
Leg, roasted, lean & fat	3 oz	230
lean only	3 oz	180
Light cure, roasted, lean & fat	3 oz	205
lean only	3 oz	135
Lunch meat, 1/8" slices	…	…
regular	2 slices	150
lean/ lowfat	2 slices	60
baked	2 slices	100
maple glazed	2 slices	120
smoked	2 slices	110
Hamburger & Cheeseburger	…	…
w/ catsup, mustard, lettuce,	…	…
& onion or pickle	…	…
4 oz burger w/o cheese	1	420
4 oz burger w/cheese	1	520
(also, see Beef- Ground	…	…
& Fast Food Restaurants)	…	…
Hamburger Helper	…	…
Beef Pasta	1 cup	270
Beef Romanoff	1 cup	290
Beef Taco	1 cup	310
Beef Teriyaki	1 cup	290
Cheesy Shells	1 cup	340
Fettuccini Alfredo	1 cup	310
Zesty Italian	1 cup	320
Hash Browns – see Potatoes	…	…
Hearts of Palm, canned	1 piece	9
Honey, 1 Tbsp	1 Tbsp	64
Honey, 1 cup	1 cup	1030
Honeydew Melon	…	…
Fresh, avg size 6 ½" melon,	…	…
cubed or diced	1 cup	60
wedge, 1/8 of melon	1 wedge	55
Horseradish, as prep	1 tsp	4
HOT DOG (FRANKFURTER)	…	…
Beef or Pork	1	145
Chicken or Turkey	1	115
Lowfat, any meat	1	75
Fat free, any meat	1	45

FOOD: (See Beverages & Restaurants listed separately)	Serving Size	Calories
Hot Dog (meal as prep)	…	…
Hot Dog on Bun	…	…
w/ catsup & mustard	1 avg	245
Hot Dog on Bun w/ chili	1 avg	295
Corndog	1 avg	395
Hummus, commercial	1 Tbsp	23
Hush Puppies	5	260
Ice Cream	…	…
Chocolate	…	…
regular	½ cup	145
reduced fat	½ cup	100
Vanilla	…	…
regular	½ cup	135
reduced fat	½ cup	90
rich	½ cup	180
soft ice cream in cone	1 cone	200
soft in cone, chocolate dipped	1 cone	255
Sherbet, Orange	½ cup	100
Ice Cream Cone, 2 ½" cup only	1 cup	20
Ice Cream Sandwich, vanilla	1	220
Ice Pop - See Frozen Dessert	…	…
Italian Ices	½ cup	65
Italian Seasoning, dried spice	½ tsp	3
Jalapeno – see Peppers	…	…
Jam	…	…
All flavors, regular	1 Tbsp	55
All flavors, restaurant packet	1 pkt	39
Jello – see Gelatin	…	…
Jelly	…	…
All flavors, regular	1 Tbsp	54
All flavors, restaurant packet	1 pkt	40
Kale	…	…
Fresh, raw	1 cup	17
Fresh, chopped, cooked	1 cup	36
Frozen, chopped, cooked	1 cup	39
Ketchup, regular	1 Tbsp	18
restaurant size packet	1 pkt	10
Kiwi fruit, fresh, medium size	1	45
Knockwurst, beef, Boars Head	1 wurst	310
Kohlrabi, cooked, slices	1 cup	48

FOOD: (See Beverages & Restaurants listed separately)	Serving Size	Calories
Lamb	...	...
(Braised, broiled, or roasted)	...	...
Arm chop, lean & fat	3 oz	295
lean only	3 oz	235
Leg of lamb, lean & fat	3 oz	220
lean only	3 oz	160
Loin chop, lean & fat	3 oz	270
lean only	3 oz	185
Rib roast, lean & fat	3 oz	305
lean only	3 oz	195
Lard, 1 cup	1 cup	1850
Lard, 1 Tbsp	1 Tbsp	115
Lasagna, avg size 2 ½" x 4 "	...	...
w/ meat sauce	1	360
w/ zucchini	1	330
Leek, chopped, cooked	1 cup	32
Lemon, fresh, 2 ¼" dia	1	20
Lentil, cooked	½ cup	115
Lettuce, fresh, raw	...	...
Bibb, Boston, Butterhead	...	...
whole head, 5" dia	1 head	21
single leaf	1 leaf	1
Iceberg, Crisphead	...	.
whole head, 6" dia	1 head	65
single leaf	1 leaf	1
pieces, chopped or shredded	1 cup	8
wedge slice, 1/6 of 6" head	1 wedge	11
Loose leaf	...	...
single leaf	1 leaf	2
pieces, shredded or chopped	1 cup	10
Romaine or cos	...	...
innerleaf	1 leaf	1
pieces, shredded	1 cup	8
Lime, fresh, 2" dia	1	20
Linguini w/Clam sauce	...	...
Lean Cuisine entrée	1 meal	260
Liver	...	...
Beef liver, fried	3 oz	185
Chicken liver, simmered	1 liver	31
Veal liver, braised	3.5 oz	165
Liverwurst, Boars Head	2 oz	170

FOOD: (See Beverages & Restaurants listed separately)	Serving Size	Calories
Lobster – see Fish / Seafood	…	…
Lo Mein w/Vegetables	1 ½ cup	230
Lo Mein w/meat & vegetables	1 ½ cup	310
Lunch Meat (thin 1/8" slices)	…	…
Beef or Pork, regular	2 slices	180
Beef or Pork, lowfat	2 slices	110
Beef or Pork, fat free	2 slices	60
Chicken or Turkey , regular	2 slices	160
Chicken or Turkey, lowfat	2 slices	100
Chicken or Turkey, fat free	2 slices	60
Ham, regular	2 slices	150
Ham, lean/lowfat	2 slices	60
(also see specific listings)	…	…
Macaroni, elbows	…	…
Dry, uncooked	1 cup	420
Plain, cooked	1 cup	195
Macaroni & Cheese	1 cup	300
Mackerel – see Fish	…	…
Malt O Meal, as prep	1 cup	122
Mandarin Oranges	…	…
Canned in light syrup	1 cup	154
Mango	…	…
Fresh, peeled, 11 oz	1	135
Fresh, peeled, sliced	1 cup	105
Manicotti, 3 cheese	2 piece	300
Margarine	…	…
Regular, 4 sticks/Lb	1 stick	815
Regular, hard or soft	1 cup	1625
Regular, hard or soft	1 Tbsp	100
Regular, hard or soft	1 tsp	34
Reduced fat 50%	1 cup	1235
Reduced fat 50%	1 tsp	25
Fat free	1 cup	512
Fat free	1 Tbsp	5
Spread or blend type, regular	1 Tbsp	100
Spread or blend w/ vegetable oil	…	…
& margarine, 33% reduced fat	1 Tbsp	60
Marjoram, dried spice	1 tsp	2
Marmalade	1 Tbsp	50
Marshmallow	…	…
Miniature size	1 cup	160

FOOD: (See Beverages & Restaurants listed separately)	Serving Size	Calories
Regular size	2 piece	46
Regular or Large size	1 oz	90
Marshmallow Topping	1 Tbsp	50
Mayonnaise	…	…
Regular	1 Tbsp	100
Light / reduced calorie	1 Tbsp	50
Fat free	1 Tbsp	10
Meat – see specific listings	…	…
Meat Tenderizer	¼ tsp	0
Meatless Burger	…	…
Single patty, broiled	1 patty	100
Cooked, crumbled	1 cup	230
Meatloaf	…	…
Banquet entrée	1 meal	280
Healthy Choice entrée	1 meal	320
Lean Cuisine entrée	1 meal	260
Meatloaf & cheese sandwich	1	350
Minestrone – see Soup	…	…
Molasses, blackstrap, 1 Tbsp	1 Tbsp	47
Molasses, blackstrap, 1 cup	1 cup	771
Mortadella	1 slice	50
Muffin	…	…
Avg size muffin, 2 ½" dia	…	…
Apple muffin	1	160
Banana muffin	1	165
Blueberry muffin	1	160
Bran w/ raisins	1	175
Chocolate Chip muffin	1	180
Corn muffin	1	175
Extra large muffin, 4" dia	…	…
Banana nut muffin	1	420
Bran w/raisins	1	425
(also see English Muffin)	…	…
Mulberries	½ cup	30
Mushroom	…	…
Regular Mushrooms	…	…
Fresh, raw, slices	1 cup	18
Fresh, sliced, cooked	1 cup	42
Canned, stems & pieces,	…	…
cooked	1 cup	37
Shiitake Mushrooms	…	…

FOOD: (See Beverages & Restaurants listed separately)	Serving Size	Calories
Dried, cut pieces, cooked	1 cup	80
Dried, whole, cooked	1 whole	11
Mussels – see Fish/Seafood	...	...
Mustard, yellow	...	...
Regular	1 tsp	4
Hot or Honey flavored	1 tsp	8
Powder	1 tsp	10
Mustard Greens, chopped, cooked	1 cup	21

FOOD: (See Beverages & Restaurants listed separately)	Serving Size	Calories
Nachos w/ Cheese sauce	7 pc	345
Nectarine, fresh, med, 2 ½" dia	1	67
Noodles (egg noodles)	...	...
Dry, uncooked	1 cup	420
Plain, cooked	1 cup	195
Chow Mein noodles,	...	...
dry crunchy	1 cup	235
Spinach noodles, cooked	1 cup	210
Noodles Alfredo	¾ cup	250
Noodles Stroganoff	¾ cup	220
Nut Pastry Filling	1 Tbsp	65
Nuts	...	...
Almonds	...	...
sliced almonds	1 cup	550
whole almonds, about 24	1 oz	165
Brazil nuts, shelled, 6 to 8 nuts	1 oz	185
Cashews	...	...
dry roasted, about 20	1 oz	160
oil roasted, about 18	1 oz	165
Chestnuts, roasted, shelled	1 cup	350
Coconut	...	...
fresh, shredded	1 cup	285
dried, sweetened flakes	1 cup	465
Hazelnuts, chopped, ¼ cup	1 oz	180
Macadamia, dry roasted, 11 nuts	1 oz	205

FOOD: (See Beverages & Restaurants listed separately)	Serving Size	Calories
Mixed Nuts w/ peanuts	...	...
dry roasted, about 20 nuts	1 oz	168
oil roasted, about 20 nuts	1 oz	175
Peanuts	...	...
dry roasted, unsalted	1 cup	855
dry roasted, unsalted, about 28	1 oz	165
dry roasted, salted, about 28	1 oz	165
honey roasted, about 28	1 oz	165
oil roasted, salted, about 26	1 oz	170
Pecans, 10 whole or 20 halves	1 oz	195
Pine nuts, shelled	1 oz	160
Pistachio nuts, dry roasted, shelled, about 47	... 1 oz	... 160
Walnuts, English	...	...
chopped	1 cup	785
whole, 7 walnuts	1 oz	185
Oat Bran	...	...
Uncooked	1 cup	230
Cooked	1 cup	88
Oatmeal, as prep	...	...
Plain, sweetened	½ cup	75
Fruit flavored oatmeal	1 pkt	135
Maple & brown sugar oatmeal	1 pkt	130
Oats, dry, 100% rolled oats	½ cup	150
OIL (for cooking & salads)	...	...
Cooking spray, ¼ second spray	1 spray	0
Canola oil	1 cup	1925
Canola oil	Tbsp	120
Corn oil	1 cup	1925
Corn oil	Tbsp	120
Cottonseed/soybean oil blend	1 cup	1925
Cottonseed/soybean oil blend	1 Tbsp	120
Olive oil	1 cup	1905
Olive oil	1 Tbsp	119
Peanut oil	1 cup	1905
Peanut oil	1 Tbsp	119
Safflower oil	1 cup	1925
Safflower oil	1 Tbsp	120
Sesame oil	1 cup	1925
Sesame oil	1 Tbsp	120
Soybean oil	1 cup	1925

FOOD: (See Beverages & Restaurants listed separately)	Serving Size	Calories
Soybean oil	1 Tbsp	120
Sunflower oil	1 cup	1925
Sunflower oil	1 Tbsp	120
Vegetable oil	1 cup	1925
Vegetable oil	1 Tbsp	120
Okra	…	…
Fresh, sliced, cooked	1 cup	51
Frozen, slices, cooked	1 cup	52
Whole, 3" pods, cooked	8 pods	30
Fried, breaded	½ cup	165
Olive	…	…
Pickled, green, medium size	5	20
Ripe, black, large size	5	25
Olive Loaf	2 oz	130
Onion	…	…
Round yellow or white onion	…	…
Fresh, raw, whole, 2 ½" dia	1 whole	42
Fresh, chopped	1 cup	61
Fresh, sliced, 1/8" thick	1 slice	5
Cooked, whole, 2 ½" dia	1 whole	41
Cooked, sliced or chopped	1 cup	92
Sprigs w/green tops & bulbs	…	…
Whole w/top, raw, chopped	1 whole	8
Bulbs only, chopped	1 cup	32
Onion Flakes, dried	1 Tbsp	16
Onion Powder or Salt	1 tsp	7
Onion Rings	…	…
Breaded, fried	5 rings	125
Orange	…	…
Fresh, medium size, 3" dia	1	70
Fresh, sections	1 cup	85
Oregano, ground	1 tsp	5
Pam, non-stick cooking spray	…	…
¼ second spray	1 spray	0
Pancake, 4" dia	…	…
Regular, toaster type	1	82
Lowfat, toaster type	1	70
Regular, from mix or scratch	1	90
Blueberry, mix or toaster type	1	85
Pancake Syrup - see Syrup	…	…

FOOD: (See Beverages & Restaurants listed separately)	Serving Size	Calories
Papaya	...	...
Fresh, peeled, 5" long x 3" dia	1	120
Fresh, peeled, cubed	1 cup	55
Paprika, dried powder	1 tsp	6
Parsley	...	...
Fresh, raw, chopped	10	4
Dried parsley bits	1 Tbsp	4
Parsnip, sliced, cooked	1 cup	125
Passion Fruit, raw, avg size	1	17
Pasta	...	...
Plain, cooked	1 cup	195
W/cheese & tomato sauce	1 cup	250
W/meatballs in tomato sauce	1 cup	260
W/shrimp & herb sauce	1 cup	295
W/tomato sauce	1 cup	240
Pasta Roni	...	...
Pasta w/broccoli	1 cup	240
Pasta w/broccoli & chicken	1 cup	260
Pasta Alfredo Primavera	1 cup	280
Pasta, Angel Hair	...	...
Prep w/herb sauce	1 cup	280
Weight Watchers entrée	1 meal	170
Pasta, Bowtie w/tomato sauce	1 cup	240
Pasta Marsala	1 cup	280
Pasta Salad w/dressing	1 cup	250
Pastrami	...	...
Regular	2 oz	90
Turkey	2 oz	60
Pastry - see Danish Pastry & specific listings	... ...	... ...
Pastry Filling -see specific listing	...	...
Peach	...	...
Fresh, whole, med, 2 ½" dia	1	42
Fresh, sliced	1 cup	76
Canned, in heavy syrup	1 cup	195
Canned, in light syrup	1 cup	150
Canned, in juice	1 cup	115
Dried, halves,	3 halves	93
Frozen, sweetened slices, thawed	1 cup	235
Peanut - see Nuts	...	...

FOOD: (See Beverages & Restaurants listed separately)	Serving Size	Calories
Peanut Butter	…	…
Regular, smooth	1 Tbsp	95
Regular, chunky	1 Tbsp	95
Reduced fat, smooth	1 Tbsp	90
Pear	…	…
Fresh, 2 ½" dia	1	50
Fresh, 3 ¼" dia	1	116
Canned, in heavy syrup	1 cup	197
Canned, in juice	1 cup	125
Peas (cooked w/o fats)	…	…
Black eyed peas	½ cup	105
Chickpeas	½ cup	140
Green peas	½ cup	60
Lentils	½ cup	115
Navy peas	½ cup	125
Pea Pods	½ cup	40
Split peas	½ cup	115
Sweet peas	½ cup	60
Peas and Carrots	½ cup	40
Pecan Pastry Filling	1 Tbsp	65
Pecans, 10 whole or 20 halves	1 oz	195
Pepper, dried powder or granules	…	…
Black	1 tsp	5
Cayenne or red	1 tsp	7
White	1 tsp	5
Pepper Steak	…	…
Stouffer's entree	1 meal	330
Le Menu entree	1 meal	354
Pepperoni, 14 thin slices/oz	1 oz	130
Peppers	…	…
Chili Peppers, hot, raw	…	…
red or green	1 whole	18
Green, sweet, raw	…	…
whole, 3" x 2 ¼"	1 whole	32
ring, ¼" thick	1 ring	3
chopped	1 cup	40
Jalapeno peppers, sliced	¼ cup	7
Red, sweet, raw	…	…
whole, 3" x 2 ¼"	1 whole	32
ring, ¼" thick	1 ring	3
chopped	1 cup	40

FOOD: (See Beverages & Restaurants listed separately)	Serving Size	Calories
Red or Green, sweet, cooked	...	...
chopped	1 cup	38
Peppers, Stuffed, Stouffers	1 cup	200
Persimmon, raw, medium size	1	32
Pickle	...	...
Bread & Butter slices, 1 ½" dia	6 slices	36
Dill, whole, 3 ¾" long	1	12
Sweet Gherkin, 2 ½" long	1	20
Pickle Relish	1 Tbsp	20
Pie (1/8 of 9" pie unless noted)	...	...
Apple pie, 2 crust	1 slice	420
Blueberry pie, 2 crust	1 slice	360
Boston Cream Pie, 1 crust	1 slice	230
Cherry pie, 2 crust	1 slice	485
Cherry, fried pie, 4" x 2"	1 slice	405
Chocolate chip pie, 1 crust	1 slice	590
Chocolate Cream pie, 1 crust	1 slice	405
Coconut Custard pie, 1 crust	1 slice	305
Lemon Meringue pie, 1 crust	1 slice	360
Peach pie, 2 crust	1 slice	410
Pecan pie, 1 crust	1 slice	505
Pumpkin pie, 1 crust	1 slice	320
Strawberry pie, 2 crust	1 slice	360
Pie Crust, 9" dia	...	...
Regular from recipe or frozen	1 crust	800
Graham cracker crust	1 crust	950
Reduced fat crust	1 crust	605
Pilaf - see Rice Pilaf	...	...
Pimiento	1 oz	10
Pineapple	...	...
Fresh, diced or sliced	1 cup	76
Canned, in heavy syrup,	...	...
chunks or crushed	1 cup	198
slices, 3" dia	1 slice	38
Canned, in juice,	...	...
chunks or crushed	1 cup	150
slices, 3" dia	1 slice	28
PIZZA (Listings for an avg size	...	...
slice, 1/8 of 12" pizza)	...	...
Thin & Crispy Pizza	...	...
Cheese	1 slice	140

FOOD: (See Beverages & Restaurants listed separately)	Serving Size	Calories
Pepperoni & Cheese	1 slice	180
One Meat w/ Vegetables	1 slice	185
Three Meat w/ Vegetables	1 slice	210
Thick & Chewy or Pan Pizza	...	...
Cheese	1 slice	270
Pepperoni & Cheese	1 slice	310
One Meat w/ Vegetables	1 slice	320
Three Meat w/ Vegetables	1 slice	405
Stuffed Crust Pizza, thick	...	...
Pepperoni & Cheese	1 slice	350
Three Meat w/ Vegetables	1 slice	450
Pizza Rolls, 1 ½", frozen, heated	...	...
With cheese and meat	5	175
Plantain, without peel	...	...
Fresh, medium size	1	218
Cooked, slices	1 cup	180
Plum	...	...
Fresh, whole, med, 2 ¼" dia	1	36
Canned, in heavy syrup	1 cup	230
Canned, in juice	1 cup	146
Pomegranate, avg size, raw	1	105
Pop Tart – see Toaster Pastry	...	...
Popcorn	...	...
Air popped	1 cup	30
Caramel coated w/ peanuts	1 cup	170
Caramel coated w/o peanuts	1 cup	150
Cheese flavored	1 cup	60
Microwave, butter flavor	1 cup	40
Microwave, butter, reduced fat	1 cup	30
Popped in oil	1 cup	55
Popped in oil, buttered	1 cup	75
Popcorn Cake, plain	1	38
Butter flavor	1	40
Carmel	1	48
Poppyseed pastry filling	1 Tbsp	65
Popsicle – see Frozen Dessert	...	...
PORK	...	...
(Weights for meat w/o bones)	...	...
Bacon, regular	3 slices	110
Bacon, Canadian	3 slices	125
Boston Butt, roasted, lean	3 oz	205

FOOD: (See Beverages & Restaurants listed separately)	Serving Size	Calories
Picnic Pork	3.5 oz	280
Pork Chop, loin cut	…	…
broiled, lean & fat	3 oz	205
broiled, lean only	3 oz	170
pan fried, lean & fat	3 oz	235
pan fried, lean only	3 oz	195
Rib Roast, lean & fat	3 oz	215
lean only	3 oz	195
Sausage	…	…
breakfast link, small	1 link	70
breakfast patty, small	1 patty	80
sausage, regular	2 oz	120
sausage, lowfat	2 oz	80
Polish Kielbasa sausage	2 oz	120
Vienna sausage, 2" links	2 links	90
Shoulder cut, braised, lean & fat	3 oz	280
lean only	3 oz	210
Spareribs, braised	3 oz	335
(Other Pork Products, see:	…	…
Bologna, Ham, Hot Dog,	…	…
Salami, & specific entrées)	…	…
Pork Chop, fried	3 oz	235
Marie Callendar entrée	1 meal	550
Pork Rinds, about 1 cup	1 oz	155
Pot Pie, 4" dia, frozen, heated	…	…
Beef Pot Pie	1 pie	480
Chicken Pot Pie	1 pie	410
Turkey Pot Pie	1 pie	400
Pot Roast	…	…
Lean Cuisine entrée	1 meal	190
Marie Callender entrée	1 meal	250
Swanson entrée	1 meal	405
POTATO	…	…
(also see Sweet Potatoes)	…	…
Au Gratin Potatoes	1 cup	300
Baked potato, 4 ¾" x 2 ¼"	…	…
whole potato w/skin	1	220
whole potato w/o skin	1	145
Baked, & filled or topped,	…	…
large potato, 6" x 2 ½"	…	…
bacon & cheese	1	530

FOOD: (See Beverages & Restaurants listed separately)	Serving Size	Calories
broccoli & cheese	1	470
cheese	1	570
chili & cheese	1	620
sour cream & chives	1	390
Boiled potato, 2 ½" dia	...	...
peeled, whole potato	1	116
peeled, diced	1 cup	134
French Fries	...	...
Frozen, heated	...	...
thin shoestring strips, 3 oz	20 fries	130
thick or crinkle cut, 4.5 oz	20 fries	195
Restaurant type, medium order	1 med	350
Hash Browns, patty, 3" x 2"	1 patty	80
Hash Browned potatoes	1 cup	280
Mashed, w/milk & margarine	1 cup	220
Scalloped potatoes	1 cup	245
Tater Tots type fried potatoes	10 pc	175
Potato Chips	...	...
(about 14 chips, unless noted)	...	...
Plain, regular	1 oz	155
Barbecue flavor	1 oz	155
Cheddar cheese	1 oz	160
Fat free chips	1 oz	75
Pringles, regular	1 oz	160
Reduced fat chips	1 oz	140
Rippled chips (about 12 chips)	1 oz	160
Ruffles, original (12 chips)	1 oz	160
Ruffles, reduced fat (13 chips)	1 oz	140
Ranch flavor chips	1 oz	155
Sour cream & onion flavor	1 oz	155
Potato Salad	1 cup	360
Potato Sticks, fried, crunchy	1 cup	250
Preserves	...	...
All flavors, regular	1 Tbsp	55
All flavors, restaurant packet	1 pkt	39
Pretzels	...	...
Sticks, regular	25	58
Mini Twists, regular	10	58
Bavarian, twisted, 2 ½" x 3"	1	60
Chocolate coated	1 oz	130
Dutch, twisted, 2 ½" x 3"	1	60

FOOD: (See Beverages & Restaurants listed separately)	Serving Size	Calories
Honey Mustard nuggets	10	150
Soft, twisted, large, 3" x 5"	1	180
Sourdough, twisted, 2 ½" x 3"	1	60
Prosciutto, Boars Head	1 oz	60
Prunes, dried, pitted	…	…
Uncooked, unsweetened	5 prunes	100
Stewed, unsweetened	1 cup	265
Pudding	…	…
Butterscotch, regular	½ cup	150
Caramel w/chocolate, regular	½ cup	150
Chocolate, regular	½ cup	150
fat free	½ cup	105
sugar free	½ cup	110
Rice pudding, regular	½ cup	185
Tapioca, regular	½ cup	135
fat free	½ cup	100
Vanilla, regular	½ cup	145
fat free	½ cup	105
sugar free	½ cup	110
Pumpkin	…	…
Fresh, cooked, mashed	1 cup	50
Canned, heated	1 cup	83
Quesadilla	…	…
Cheese	1	350
Chicken	1	400
Radish, fresh, raw, avg 1" dia	5	5
Raisin	…	…
Golden or natural, not packed	1 cup	435
Golden or natural, 0.5 oz pkg	1 pkg	42
Golden or natural, not packed	3 Tbsp	84
Raisin Bran – see Cereal	…	…
Raspberries	…	…
Fresh	1 cup	60
Frozen, sweetened, thawed	1 cup	260
Ravioli	…	…
Beef	1 cup	255
Cheese	1 cup	265
Relish – see Pickle Relish or specific listing	… …	… …
Rhubarb	…	…
Fresh, diced	1 cup	28

FOOD: (See Beverages & Restaurants listed separately)	Serving Size	Calories
Frozen, cooked, sweetened	1 cup	278
RICE	...	...
Plain Rice Dishes	...	...
Brown long grain rice, boiled	1 cup	215
Brown long grain, prep w/butter	1 cup	315
Long grain & wild rice, boiled	1 cup	200
Long grain & wild prep w/butter	1 cup	300
White rice, boiled	1 cup	200
White rice, prep w/butter	1 cup	300
Wild rice, boiled	1 cup	170
Wild rice, prep w/butter	1 cup	270
Yellow rice, boiled	1 cup	220
Mixed & Flavored Rice Dishes	...	...
Flavored w/ beef or pork	1 cup	280
Fried rice w/ beef	1 cup	295
Fried rice w/ chicken	1 cup	265
Fried rice w/ pork	1 cup	290
Fried rice w/ shrimp	1 cup	260
Fried rice w/ vegetables	1 cup	255
Rice & beans	1 cup	300
Rice & vegetables	1 cup	260
Rice Pilaf w/vegetables	1 cup	240
Rice-a-Roni	...	...
Beef vermicelli rice dish	1 cup	290
Broccoli & cheddar rice dish	1 cup	330
Cheddar & herbs rice dish	1 cup	310
Chicken & vegetable rice	1 cup	290
Chicken vermicelli rice dish	1 cup	290
Herb & butter rice dish	1 cup	280
Mexican style rice	1 cup	265
Rice pilaf	1 cup	305
Spanish rice dish	1 cup	270
Rice Cake, plain	1	35
Butter flavor	1	40
Carmel	1	48
Rice Krispies Treat	1 bar	90
Rigatoni, meat sauce	...	...
Lean Cuisine entrée	1 meal	260
Roast Beef – see Beef	...	...
Roast Beef Sandwich	...	...
3 oz meat w/ sauce	1 avg	390

FOOD: (See Beverages & Restaurants listed separately)	Serving Size	Calories
Rolls – see Bread	…	…
Rosemary, dried spice	½ tsp	2
Rutabaga, cubed, cooked	1 cup	65
Saccharin sweetener	1 pkt	0
Sage, dried spice	½ tsp	1
SALAD DRESSING	…	…
Blue cheese, regular	1 Tbsp	75
Blue cheese, low calorie	1 Tbsp	15
Buttermilk, regular	1 Tbsp	60
Buttermilk, low calorie	1 Tbsp	15
Caesar, regular	1 Tbsp	80
Caesar, low calorie	1 Tbsp	17
French, regular	1 Tbsp	70
French, low calorie	1 Tbsp	25
Honey Dijon, regular	1 Tbsp	70
Honey Dijon, fat free	1 Tbsp	25
Italian, regular	1 Tbsp	70
Italian, low calorie	1 Tbsp	16
Mayonnaise, regular	1 Tbsp	100
Mayonnaise, light	1 Tbsp	50
Mayonnaise, fat free	1 Tbsp	10
Ranch, regular	1 Tbsp	70
Ranch, low calorie	1 Tbsp	20
Russian, regular	1 Tbsp	75
Russian, low calorie	1 Tbsp	25
Thousand island, regular	1 Tbsp	65
Thousand island, low calorie	1 Tbsp	26
Zero Carb Salad Dressing	…	…
Nature's Flavors	…	…
Carbfree Blue Cheese	2 Tbsp	30
Carbfree French	2 Tbsp	30
Salad, Tossed	…	…
All Vegetable salad, no dressing	1 ½ cup	60
Salad w/egg & cheese	…	…
no dressing	1 ½ cup	120
w/regular dressing, any type	1 ½ cup	200
w/light dressing, any type	1 ½ cup	135
Salad w/grilled chicken or turkey	…	…
no dressing	1 ½ cup	150
w/regular dressing, any type	1 ½ cup	250
w/light dressing, any type	1 ½ cup	175

FOOD: (See Beverages & Restaurants listed separately)	Serving Size	Calories
(Also see Pasta Salad, Potato Salad, & specific listings)	... ...	... ...
Salami	...	...
Regular, any meat	2 oz	130
Lowfat, Turkey or Chicken,	...	...
thin 1/8" slices	2 slices	80
Cotto	2 slices	95
Dried type, 3" x 1/8" slices	2 slices	95
Hard	1 oz	110
Salisbury Steak	...	...
Banquet entrée	1 meal	220
Morton's entrée	1 meal	210
Stouffer's entrée	1 meal	240
Weight Watchers entrée	1 meal	150
Salsa	1 Tbsp	4
Salt	...	...
Regular	½ tsp	0
Reduced sodium	½ tsp	0
Seasoned	½ tsp	5
Sandwich, (w/ 3 oz Meat on Lg 6" bun, sub, or kaiser roll)	... ...	... ...
Cold Cuts, mixed meats w/	...	...
sauce, cheese, tomato, lettuce	1	455
Ham & Cheese w/ sauce	1	495
Roast Beef w/ mayo, tomato,	...	...
lettuce	1	498
Tuna salad w/ mayo, lettuce	1	585
Sandwich Meat, see Lunch Meat	...	...
Sandwich Spread	1 Tbsp	35
SAUCE	...	...
A1 Steak Sauce	1 Tbsp	15
Barbecue sauce, regular	1 Tbsp	20
Barbecue, thick or honey	1 Tbsp	40
Catsup	1 Tbsp	18
Cheese sauce	¼ cup	110
Chili sauce	¼ cup	60
Duck Sauce	1 Tbsp	20
Hoison sauce	1 Tbsp	35
Hollandaise sauce	1 Tbsp	18
Horseradish, prepared	1 tsp	4
Hot sauce	1 tsp	1

FOOD: (See Beverages & Restaurants listed separately)	Serving Size	Calories
Marinara sauce	¼ cup	36
Mayonnaise, regular	1 Tbsp	100
Mayonnaise, light	1 Tbsp	50
Mayonnaise, fat free	1 Tbsp	10
Mustard, regular	1 tsp	4
Mustard, hot or honey	1 tsp	8
Oyster sauce	1 Tbsp	5
Pasta sauce	¼ cup	35
Pepper sauce, hot	1 tsp	1
Pickle Relish	1 Tbsp	20
Pizza sauce	¼ cup	35
Salsa	1 Tbsp	4
Sloppy Joe sauce w/meat	1 Tbsp	45
Soy sauce	1 Tbsp	10
Spaghetti sauce	¼ cup	36
Steak Sauce	1 Tbsp	15
Sweet & Sour Sauce	1 Tbsp	20
Szechuan sauce	1 Tbsp	20
Tabasco sauce	1 tsp	1
Taco sauce	1 Tbsp	10
Tamari Sauce	1 Tbsp	11
Tartar sauce	1 Tbsp	45
Teriyaki sauce	1 Tbsp	20
Tomato sauce	½ cup	37
White sauce	¼ cup	92
Worcestershire sauce	1 Tbsp	12
Zero Carb Sauce	…	…
Nature's Flavors	…	…
Barbecue sauce	2 Tbsp	0
Honey Mustard sauce	2 Tbsp	0
Sauerkraut	1 cup	45
Sausage	…	…
Breakfast link, small	1 link	70
Breakfast patty, small	1 patty	80
Beef or Pork sausage	2 oz	120
Chicken or Turkey sausage	2 oz	98
Lowfat sausage, beef or pork	2 oz	80
Lowfat sausage,chicken or turkey	2 oz	78
Fat free sausage, beef or pork	2 oz	60
Fat free sausage, chicken or turkey	… 2 oz	… 58

FOOD: (See Beverages & Restaurants listed separately)	Serving Size	Calories
Polish sausage, Kielbasa	2 oz	120
Vienna sausage, 2" links	2 links	90
Scallop - see Fish/Seafood	...	...
Seafood – see Fish/Seafood	...	...
Seasoning – see specific listings	...	...
Blended Seasoning w/ salt,	...	...
garlic, onion, paprika, papain	½ tsp	2
Seaweed	...	...
Kelp, raw	2 Tbsp	4
Spirulina, dried	1 Tbsp	3
Thin wrap sheets	1 sheet	10
Seeds	...	...
Pumpkin seeds, roasted	1 oz	148
Sesame seeds, plain	1 Tbsp	47
Sesame seeds, butter, roasted	1 Tbsp	90
Soybean seeds, dried, boiled	½ cup	145
Sunflower seeds, dry roasted	1 oz	165
(Also see specific listings)	...	...
Shallot, raw, chopped	1 Tbsp	7
Shark – see Fish	...	...
Sherbet, Orange	½ cup	100
Sherbet, Rainbow	½ cup	105
Shortening, regular cottonseed &	1 cup	1810
soybean blend	1 Tbsp	115
Shrimp – see Fish/Seafood	...	...
& specific entrées	...	...
Shrimp & Broccoli	...	...
w/creamy white sauce	1 cup	270
Shrimp & Pasta	...	...
w/creamy white sauce	1 cup	300
Shrimp & Vegetables	...	...
Hunan style	1 cup	240
Shrimp & Vegetables	...	...
w/szechuan sauce	1 cup	230
Shrimp Marinara	...	...
Weight Watchers entrée	1 meal	200
Sirloin Steak – see Beef	...	...
Snack Mix, Chex Mix	¾ cup	120
Sorbet, orange or raspberry	½ cup	120
Soufflé, regular type	1 cup	250

FOOD: (See Beverages & Restaurants listed separately)	Serving Size	Calories
SOUP (as prep)	…	…
Bouillon cube, regular,	…	…
all varieties, makes 1 cup	1 cube	5
Bouillon packet, low sodium,	…	…
all varieties, makes 1 cup	1 pkt	15
Broth, consommé, all varieties	1 cup	20
Bean w/ Ham soup	1 cup	185
Bean w/ Pork soup	1 cup	175
Beef Noodle soup	1 cup	83
Chicken Noodle soup, regular	1 cup	75
Chicken Noodle soup, chunky	1 cup	175
Chicken & Rice soup	1 cup	70
Chicken & Vegetable, regular	1 cup	90
Chicken & Vegetable, chunky	1 cup	165
Clam Chowder, Manhattan	1 cup	85
Clam Chowder, New England	1 cup	165
Clam Chowder, Low fat,	…	…
New England	1 cup	115
Cream of Broccoli soup	…	…
prep w/ water	1 cup	125
prep w/ milk	1 cup	195
Cream of Chicken soup	…	…
prep w/ water	1 cup	117
prep w/ milk	1 cup	190
Cream of Mushroom soup	…	…
prep w/ water	1 cup	130
prep w/ milk	1 cup	200
Lentil soup, low fat	1 cup	125
Minestrone	1 cup	85
Onion soup	1 cup	100
Pea soup	1 cup	160
Potato w/ bean soup	1 cup	170
Ramen Beef Noodle soup	1 cup	190
Ramen Chicken noodle soup	1 cup	190
Ramen Mushroom noodle soup	1 cup	180
Tomato soup, prep w/ water	1 cup	85
Tomato soup, prep w/ milk	1 cup	160
Vegetable soup	1 cup	72
Vegetable Beef soup	1 cup	90
Wisconsin Cheese soup	1 cup	280
Sour cream	…	…

FOOD: (See Beverages & Restaurants listed separately)	Serving Size	Calories
Regular	1 cup	495
Regular	1 Tbsp	25
Reduced fat	1 Tbsp	20
Fat free	1 Tbsp	12
Soy Burger, broiled	1 patty	100
Soybeans	…	…
dried mature seeds, cooked	½ cup	145
Spaghetti	…	…
Plain, cooked	1 cup	195
With cheese & tomato sauce	1 cup	220
With meatballs in tomato sauce	1 cup	240
With tomato sauce	1 cup	260
Spaghetti Bolognese, w/ meat sauce, Healthy Choice entrée	… 1 meal	… 255
Spare Ribs – see Pork	…	…
Spice – see specific listings	…	…
Blended Spice w/ basil, garlic, oregano, rosemary, thyme	… ½ tsp	… 3
Spinach	…	…
Fresh, raw, chopped	1 cup	7
Fresh, chopped, cooked	1 cup	41
Frozen, chopped, cooked	1 cup	53
Canned, cooked	1 cup	50
Spinach Soufflé	1 cup	220
Spread	…	…
Cheese Spread	1 Tbsp	40
Sandwich Spread	1 Tbsp	35
(also see spreads in Margarine)	…	…
Squash	…	…
Butternut squash	¾ cup	150
Summer, raw, sliced	1 cup	23
Summer, cooked, slices	1 cup	36
Winter, baked, cubes	1 cup	80
Winter, frozen, cooked, mashed	1 cup	94
Squash Casserole	¾ cup	330
Steak – see Beef	…	…
Steak Sauce, A1	1 Tbsp	15
Strawberries	…	…
Fresh, medium size, 1 ¼" dia	10	40
Fresh, sliced	1 cup	50

FOOD: (See Beverages & Restaurants listed separately)	Serving Size	Calories
Frozen, sweetened, thawed	1 cup	245
Strawberry Shortcake	1 avg	275
Streusel (avg size slice)	…	…
Apple	1 slice	240
Cherry	1 slice	205
Stuffing, as prep	…	…
Traditional stuffing, seasoned,	…	…
meat flavored	1 cup	360
Corn bread stuffing, seasoned	1 cup	345
Succotash	½ cup	80
Sugar	…	…
White, regular, granulated	…	…
One cup	1 cup	774
One tablespoon	1 Tbsp	45
One teaspoon	1 tsp	15
Restaurant size packet	1 pkt	24
White, Confectioner's, Powdered	…	…
Unsifted, one cup	1 cup	31
Unsifted, one tablespoon	1 Tbsp	467
Brown Sugar	…	…
Packed, one cup	1 cup	827
Not packed , one cup	1 cup	545
Not packed, one tablespoon	1 Tbsp	34
Sugar Substitute	…	…
Aspartame – Equal, Nutrasweet	1 pkt	0
Saccharine - Sweet & Low	1 pkt	0
Sucralose - Splenda	1 pkt	0
Sundae (small serving)	…	…
Hot Fudge	1	285
Strawberry	1	230
Strawberry Yogurt	1	275
Swedish Meatballs	…	…
Celentano, 6 meatball meal	1 meal	260
Lean Cuisine entrée	1 meal	290
Weight Watchers entrée	1 meal	290
Sweet 'N Low	1 pkt	0
Sweet Potato	…	…
Baked w/skin 4" x 2"	1 whole	165
Baked or Boiled w/o skin 4" x 2"	1 whole	150
Boiled, peeled, mashed	½ cup	170

FOOD: (See Beverages & Restaurants listed separately)	Serving Size	Calories
Candied, 2 ½" x 2" pieces	1 piece	145
Canned in syrup, drained	1 cup	210
Canned, vacuum pack, mashed	1 cup	230
Whipped, frozen, heated	½ cup	140
Sweet Potato Casserole	¾ cup	280
Sweet Roll - see specific listings	...	...
Syrup	...	...
Butterscotch	1 Tbsp	60
Chocolate, thin	1 Tbsp	55
Chocolate fudge, thick	1 Tbsp	65
Corn, light	1 Tbsp	56
Maple	1 Tbsp	52
Molasses, blackstrap	1 Tbsp	47
Pancake Syrup/Table Syrup	...	...
Regular	1 Tbsp	55
Light, reduced calorie	1 Tbsp	25
Sugar free	1 Tbsp	8
Zero Carb Syrup	...	...
Nature's Flavors	...	...
Apple	2 Tbsp	0
Brown Sugar	2 Tbsp	0
Chocolate	2 Tbsp	0
Maple	1 Tbsp	0
Taco (w/hard or soft shell)	...	...
Regular size, with beef	1	210
Regular size, with chicken	1	190
Large, with steak or beef	1	280
X-Lg, double decker, with beef	1	365
Taco Salad w/ ground beef, cheese, taco shell	... 1	... 275
Taco Shell (shell only)	...	...
Thin shell, 6" dia	1	60
Large shell	1	100
Tahini, from toasted kernels	1 Tbsp	90
Tamale, meatless	2 pc	215
Beef, Swanson entrée	1 meal	350
Chicken, Swanson entrée	1 meal	325
Tangerine, fresh, med, 2 ½" dia	1	37
Tapioca, pearl, dry	1 cup	545
Taro Leaf, steamed	½ cup	18
Tarragon, ground	1 tsp	5

FOOD: (See Beverages & Restaurants listed separately)	Serving Size	Calories
Tater Tots fried potatoes	10	175
T-bone Steak – see Beef	...	...
Teriyaki – see Beef Teriyaki or Chicken Teriyaki	... ...	... ...
Thyme, dried spice	½ tsp	2
Toaster Pastry (Pop Tart)	...	...
Apple, frosted	1 pastry	200
Apple, unfrosted	1 pastry	185
Blueberry, frosted	1 pastry	200
Blueberry, unfrosted	1 pastry	185
Brown sugar, cinnamon, frosted	1 pastry	190
Chocolate, frosted	1 pastry	200
Chocolate fudge, frosted	1 pastry	200
Grape, frosted	1 pastry	200
Grape, unfrosted	1 pastry	185
Lowfat, frosted, any variety	1 pastry	170
Lowfat, unfrosted, any variety	1 pastry	155
S'mores, frosted	1 pastry	220
Strawberry, frosted	1 pastry	200
Strawberry, unfrosted	1 pastry	185
Tofu, plain, cooked, 4 oz	½ cup	80
Tomatillos, raw, medium size	2	22
Tomato	...	...
Fresh, raw, avg size 2 ½" dia	1 whole	26
Fresh, raw, cherry tomato	1 whole	4
Fresh, slices, ¼" thick	1 slice	4
Fresh, chopped or sliced	1 cup	38
Canned, liquids and solids	1 cup	46
Stewed, fresh or canned	1 cup	70
Sun Dried	...	...
Plain	1 piece	5
Packed in oil, drained	1 piece	6
Tomato Paste	1 cup	215
Tomato Puree	1 cup	100
Tomato Sauce	1 cup	74
Topping, for dessert	...	...
Butterscotch, regular	1 Tbsp	60
Butterscotch, light	1 Tbsp	30
Chocolate, regular	1 Tbsp	50
Chocolate, light	1 Tbsp	25

FOOD: (See Beverages & Restaurants listed separately)	Serving Size	Calories
Cream, Whipped Topping	…	…
Light cream	1 cup	700
Light cream	1 Tbsp	45
Heavy cream	1 cup	820
Heavy cream	1 Tbsp	50
Pressurized in can	1 Tbsp	8
Marshmallow Topping	1 Tbsp	50
Strawberry Topping	1 Tbsp	50
Tortellini	…	…
Cheese filling	1 cup	270
Meat filling	1 cup	340
Spinach filling	1 cup	235
Tortellini Salad w/dressing	¾ cup	350
Tortilla, 6" dia, ready to cook	…	…
Corn	1	60
Flour	1	105
Tortilla Chips	…	…
Regular	1 oz	140
Lowfat, baked	1 oz	115
Nacho flavor, regular	1 oz	140
Nacho flavor, reduced fat, baked	1 oz	125
(also see Corn Chips)	…	…
Tostada	…	…
Beef, bean, & cheese	1	330
Chicken & cheese	1	250
Guacamole	1	180
Trail Mix	…	…
Regular w/raisins, nuts, seeds,	…	…
& chocolate chips	1 cup	705
Tropical dried fruit mix	1 cup	570
Tuna – see Fish	…	…
Tuna Dishes	…	…
Tuna & broccoli w/creamy sauce	1 cup	300
Tuna & noodle casserole	1 cup	320
Tuna & pasta w/cheese sauce	1 cup	300
Tuna & pasta w/creamy sauce	1 cup	300
Tuna au gratin	1 cup	310
Tuna fettuccine alfredo	1 cup	310
Tuna romanoff	1 cup	280
Tuna tetrazzini	1 cup	310
Tuna Salad	…	…

FOOD: (See Beverages & Restaurants listed separately)	Serving Size	Calories
Prep w/tuna in oil, regular	...	...
mayo dressing, pickle relish	½ cup	190
Prep w/ tuna in water, light	...	...
mayo dressing, pickle relish	½ cup	130
TURKEY	...	...
Fried Turkey patty, battered	3 oz	250
Roast Turkey	...	...
light & dark meat	3 oz	145
light meat only	3 oz	135
dark meat only	3 oz	160
Giblets, simmered, chopped	1 cup	240
Ground Turkey	4 oz	195
Neck, simmered	4 oz	155
(Other Turkey Products, see:	...	...
Bologna, Hot Dog, Salami,	...	...
Sausage & specific entrées)	...	...
Turkey & Gravy	...	...
Banquet entrée	1 meal	140
Turkey Dijon	...	...
Lean Cuisine entrée	1 meal	280
Turkey Tetrazzini	...	...
Stouffers entrée	1 meal	360
Turmeric, ground	½ tsp	4
Turnip, sliced, cooked	½ cup	20
Turnip Greens, cooked	½ cup	16
Turnover	...	...
Apple or Cherry, large	1	410
Apple, small	1	170
Blueberry, small	1	165
Cherry, small	1	175
Vanilla Extract	1 tsp	12
Veal	...	...
Chop, loin, braised	3.5 oz	285
Cutlet, braised, lean & fat	3 oz	180
Liver, braised	3.5 oz	165
Rib, roasted, lean & fat	3.5 oz	250
Veal Marsala, Le Menu entrée	1 meal	250
Veal Parmagiana	...	...
Le Menu entrée	1 meal	175
Morton entrée	1 meal	280

FOOD: (See Beverages & Restaurants listed separately)	Serving Size	Calories
Vegetable Burger, broiled	1 patty	100
Vegetables, mixed	…	…
(See specific listings for	…	…
individual vegetables)	…	…
Mixed, canned, drained, heated	1 cup	80
Mixed, frozen, w/o sauce, heated	…	…
Small vegetables- peas, carrots,	…	…
beans, corn	1 cup	105
Large vegetable cuts- broccoli,	…	…
cauliflower, mushrooms	1 cup	27
Large vegetable cuts	…	…
prep w/ butter sauce	1 cup	107
Vegetables, mixed, Birdseye	…	…
French style	¾ cup	110
Italian style	½ cup	100
Japanese style	½ cup	90
Mexican style	½ cup	140
Oriental style	½ cup	60
Vinegar	…	…
Regular	1 Tbsp	2
Cider vinegar	1 Tbsp	2
Waffle	…	…
Regular, prep from recipe, 7" dia	1 piece	215
Frozen, toaster size, 4 " dia	1 piece	90
Lowfat, toaster size, 4" dia	1 piece	80
Walnut – see Nuts	…	…
Water Chestnut, canned, slices	1 cup	75
Watercress, raw	½ cup	2
Watermelon	…	…
Fresh, diced	1 cup	50
Fresh, wedge, 1" thick, 1/16 of	…	…
melon 15" long x 7 ½" dia	1 wedge	92
Wheat Bran	¼ cup	25
Wheat Germ, toasted, plain	1 Tbsp	27
Whipped Cream – see Cream	…	…
Wiener – see Hot Dog	…	…
Yam – see Sweet Potato	…	…
Yeast	…	…
Compressed	1 cake	18
Dry, active, regular size pkg	1 pkg	21

FOOD: (See Beverages & Restaurants listed separately)	Serving Size	Calories
Dry, active	1 tsp	12
Yogurt	…	…
Chocolate, regular	½ cup	120
Chocolate, fat free	½ cup	90
Strawberry, regular	½ cup	120
Strawberry, fat free	½ cup	100
Vanilla, regular	½ cup	120
Vanilla, fat free	½ cup	110
Yogurt, plain,	…	…
made w/ whole milk	½ cup	140
made w/ lowfat milk	½ cup	130
made w/ skim milk	½ cup	120
Yogurt w/fruit, regular varieties	½ cup	135
Yogurt, w/fruit flavor, sugarfree	½ cup	95
Ziti w/ Meat Sauce	…	…
Swanson entrée	1 meal	560
Zucchini	…	…
Fresh, avg size	1	5
Sliced, cooked	½ cup	15
Breaded, fried	½ cup	165

FAST FOOD RESTAURANTS

RESTAURANT: (See other Foods and Beverages listed separately)	Serving Size	Calories
Arby's	...	...
Apple turnover	1	330
Arby-Q	1	430
Arby's melt w/ cheddar	1	370
Arby's sauce	1 svg	15
Bacon cheddar deluxe	1	540
Baked potato, deluxe	1	735
Baked potato, plain	1	355
Baked potato w/sour cream	1	580
Barbecue sauce	1 svg	30
Beef & cheddar sandwich	1	490
Beefstock Au Jus	1	10
Biscuit, plain	1	280
Bleu cheese dressing	1 svg	290
Blueberry muffin	1	230
Boston clam chowder	1 svg	190
Breaded chicken fillet	1	542
Broccoli & cheddar baked potato	1	580
Butterfinger polar swirl	1	455
Cheddar cheese sauce	1 svg	35
Cheddar curly fries	1 svg	335
Cheesecake, plain	1	320
Cherry turnover	1	320
Chicken Cordon Bleu	1	625
Chicken fingers, 2 pieces/svg	1 svg	290
Chocolate chip cookie	1	125
Chocolate shake	med	450
Cinnamon nut Danish	1	360
Cream of broccoli soup	1 svg	160
Croissant, plain	1	220
Curly fries	1 svg	300
Fish fillet	1	530
French dip	1 svg	475
French fries	1	240
French toast stix, 6 pieces/svg	1 svg	430
Garden salad w/o dressing	1	60
Grilled chicken deluxe	1	430
Grilled chicken barbecue	1	390
Ham & cheese	1	355

RESTAURANT: (See other Foods and Beverages listed separately)	Serving Size	Calories
Ham & cheese melt	1	335
Heath polar swirl	1	545
Honey French dressing	1 svg	275
Horsey sauce	1 svg	55
Hot ham & Swiss	1	500
Italian sub sandwich	1	670
Italian sub sauce	1 svg	70
Jamocha shake	small	385
Junior roast beef	1	325
Light mayonnaise	1 svg	12
Lumberjack mixed vegetables	1 svg	90
Old fashion chicken noodle soup	1 svg	80
Oreo polar swirl	1	480
Parmesan cheese sauce	1 svg	70
Peanut butter cup polar swirl	1	515
Philly beef & Swiss	1	750
Potato cakes	1 svg	200
Potato with bacon soup	1 svg	170
Red ranch dressing	1 svg	75
Reduced cal honey mayonnaise	1 svg	70
Reduced calorie Italian dressing	1 svg	20
Reduced cal buttermilk ranch	1 svg	50
Roast beef sandwich, regular	1	390
Roast beef deluxe sandwich	1	300
Roast beef sub sandwich	1	700
Roast chicken club	1	545
Roast chicken Santa Fe	1	435
Roast chicken deluxe	1	280
Roast chicken salad	1	150
Roast turkey deluxe	1	260
Side salad w/o dressing	1	25
Snickers polar swirl	1	510
Super roast beef	1	525
Timberline chili	1 svg	220
Triple cheese melt	1	720
Turkey sub sandwich	1	550
Vanilla shake	small	360
Wisconsin cheese soup	1 svg	280
Baskin Robbins	…	…
Aloha berry banana smoothie	1	165
Bora berry smoothie	1	175
Café mocha yogurt	1	80

RESTAURANT: (See other Foods and Beverages listed separately)	Serving Size	Calories
Calypso berry smoothie	1	160
Chocolate chip ice cream	1	155
Chocolate chocolate chip, sugarfree	... 1	... 100
Chocolate ice cream	1	155
Chocolate yogurt	1	80
Copa banana smoothie	1	145
Daiquiri ice	1	110
Dutch chocolate	1	105
Espresso & cream	1	110
Maui brownie madness	1	145
Perils of praline	1	130
Rainbow sherbet	1	120
Raspberry cheese Louise	1	135
Red raspberry sorbet	1	120
Rocky road ice cream	1	165
Silk chocolate	1	120
Strawberry yogurt, nonfat	1	105
Sunset orange smoothie	1	150
Thin mint, sugarfree	1	100
Tropic of fruit yogurt, nonfat	1	130
Tropical tango smoothie	1	180
Vanilla bean dream yogurt, nonfat	... 1	... 110
Vanilla bean dream	1	120
Vanilla chocolate twist, nonfat	1	100
Vanilla ice cream	1	145
Vanilla yogurt	1	80
Very berry strawberry ice cream	1	120
Boston Market	...	...
Apples w/ cinnamon	1 svg	252
Barbecue baked beans	1 svg	330
Black beans with rice	1 svg	300
Broccoli and rice casserole	1svg	240
Brownie, chocolate	1	310
Cake, chocolate	1 piece	505
Cake, hummingbird	1 piece	705
Carrots, glazed	1 svg	280
Cheesecake	1 piece	575
Chicken with skin, ½	1	625
Chicken w/o skin, ¼, dark meat	1	210
Chicken with skin, ¼, dark meat	1	325

RESTAURANT: (See other Foods and Beverages listed separately)	Serving Size	Calories
Chicken w/o skin, ¼, white meat	1	165
Chicken w/ skin, ¼, white meat	1	310
Chicken Caesar salad	1	670
Chicken pot pie	1	745
Chicken salad sandwich	1	675
Chicken sandwich	1	390
Chicken sandwich, barbecued	1	540
Chicken sandwich w/cheese	1	630
Cole slaw	1 svg	300
Cookie, chocolate chip	1	390
Cookie, oatmeal	1	390
Cookie, peanut butter	1	420
Corn, buttered w/herbs	1 svg	180
Corn, whole kernel	1 svg	180
Cornbread	1 svg	200
Cranberry relish	1 svg	330
Cranberry walnut relish	1 svg	365
Green beans	1 svg	80
Green bean casserole	1 svg	85
Ham with honey glaze	5 oz	210
Ham sandwich	1	410
Ham sandwich w/cheese & sauce	1	655
Macaroni and cheese	1 svg	280
Meatloaf	5 oz	290
Meatloaf sandwich w/ cheese	1	695
Meatloaf sandwich, open faced	1	730
Pie, apple streusel	1 piece	480
Pie, cherry streusel	1 piece	410
Pie, pecan	1 piece	555
Pie, pumpkin	1 piece	370
Potatoes, dill & garlic	1 svg	130
Potatoes, mashed	1 svg	185
Potatoes, mashed w/gravy	1 svg	205
Potatoes, new	1 svg	130
Potato salad	1 svg	200
Red beans and rice	1 svg	260
Rice pilaf	1 svg	180
Salad, Caesar	1 svg	200
Salad, chunky chicken	1 svg	480
Salad, cucumber	1 svg	120
Salad, fruit	1 svg	70
Salad, tortellini	1 svg	350

RESTAURANT: (See other Foods and Beverages listed separately)	Serving Size	Calories
Spinach, creamed	1 svg	260
Squash, butternut	1 svg	160
Squash casserole	1 svg	335
Stuffing, savory	1 svg	310
Sweet potato casserole	1 svg	280
Turkey bacon club sandwich	1	780
Turkey breast w/o skin	5 oz	170
Turkey sandwich, regular	1	390
Turkey sandwich w/cheese	1	615
Turkey sandwich, open faced	1	715
Vegetables, steamed, w/o sauce	1 svg	35
Zucchini marinara	1 svg	80
Burger King	…	…
A.M. express dip	1 svg	85
A.M. express grape jam	1 svg	30
A.M. express strawberry jam	1 svg	30
Bacon bits	1 svg	15
Barbecue sauce	1 svg	35
Barbecue sauce, bull's eye	1 svg	20
Biscuit with sausage	1	585
Biscuit w/ bacon, egg & cheese	1	510
BK big fish	1	695
BK broiler	1	550
Bleu cheese dressing	1 svg	160
Broiled chicken salad	1	200
Cheeseburger	1	385
Chicken sandwich	1	705
Chicken tenders, 8 pieces/svg	1 svg	310
Chocolate shake	med	445
Croissanwich with sausage, egg & cheese	… 1	… 600
Croutons	1 svg	30
Double cheeseburger	1	605
Double cheeseburger w/ bacon	1	640
Double whopper	1	875
Double whopper w/ cheese	1	965
Dutch apple pie	1	300
French dressing	1 svg	145
French fries	med	375
French fries, coated	med	340
French toast sticks	1 svg	505
Garden salad w/o dressing	1	100

RESTAURANT: (See other Foods and Beverages listed separately)	Serving Size	Calories
Hamburger	1	335
Hash browns	1	220
Honey dressing	1 svg	90
Land o'lakes classic whip blend	1 svg	65
Onion rings	1 svg	315
Ranch dressing	1 svg	175
Reduced calorie Italian dressing	1 svg	15
Side salad w/o dressing	1	60
Strawberry shake	med	425
Sweet & sour sauce	1 svg	45
Tartar sauce	1 svg	145
Thousand island dressing	1 svg	180
Vanilla shake	med	305
Whopper junior	1	425
Whopper junior w/ cheese	1	460
Whopper	1	645
Whopper w/ cheese	1	735
Chinese Restaurant – see Panda Express Chinese Food	… …	… …
Dairy Queen (all listings regular size, unless noted)	… … …	… … …
Banana split	1	515
Buster bar	1	445
Butterfinger blizzard	1	750
Caramel & nut bar	1	260
Chocolate cone	1	360
Chocolate soft serve	½ cup	150
Chocolate dilly bar	1	450
Chocolate dilly bar, mint	1	190
Chocolate malt	1	880
Chocolate shake	1	770
Chocolate sundae	1	410
Cookie dough blizzard	1	945
Dipped cone	1	515
DQ frozen heart cake	1 piece	270
DQ frozen log cake	1 piece	280
DQ frozen round cake	1 piece	340
DQ frozen sheet cake	1 piece	350
DQ fudge bar	1	60
DQ lemon freez'r	1	80
DQ orange bar	1	60

RESTAURANT: (See other Foods and Beverages listed separately)	Serving Size	Calories
DQ sandwich	1	150
DQ vanilla orange bar	1	60
DQ vanilla soft serve	½ cup	140
DQ yogurt, nonfat frozen	½ cup	100
Fudge nut bar	1	410
Heath blizzard	1	818
Heath breeze	1	710
Heath treatzza pizza	1 slice	180
M&M treatzza pizza	1 slice	190
Misty slush	1	290
Oreo blizzard	1	640
Peanut buster parfait	1	730
Peanut butter fudge treatzza pizza	1 slice	220
Queen's choice choc. big scoop	1	250
Queen's choice vanilla big scoop	1	250
Reeses peanut butter cup blizzard	1	785
Starkiss	1	80
Strawberry blizzard	1	570
Strawberry breeze	1	460
Strawberry misty cooler	1 piece	190
Strawberry shortcake	1	430
Toffee dilly bar	1	210
Vanilla cone	1	355
Vanilla cone, small	1	230
Yogurt cone	1	280
Yogurt cup	1	230
Yogurt strawberry sundae	1	305
Denny's	…	…
Banana split	1	885
Biscuit with sausage gravy	7 oz	395
Buffalo wings, 12 per svg	1 svg	855
Carrots with honey glaze	1 svg	80
Charleston chicken dinner	1	325
Cheesecake	1 slice	470
Cheese fries with chili	1 svg	815
Cheese fries, smothered	1 svg	765
Chicken burger sandwich	1	630
Chicken burger buffalo sandwich	1	800
Chicken fried steak	4 oz	265
Chicken strips, 5 per svg	1 svg	720
Chicken strips buffalo, 5 per svg	1 svg	735
Chili with cheese topping	1 svg	400

RESTAURANT: (See other Foods and Beverages listed separately)	Serving Size	Calories
Chocolate layer cake	1 slice	275
Club sandwich	1	720
Corn with butter sauce	1 svg	120
Country fried potatoes	1 svg	515
Double scoop sundae	1	375
French fries	1 svg	260
French fries w/ seasoning	1 svg	320
Fried shrimp dinner	8 oz	220
Garden salad deluxe w/ chicken	1	265
Grasshopper blender blaster	15 oz	735
Grasshopper sundae	14 oz	735
Green beans w/ bacon	1 svg	60
Green peas w/ butter sauce	1 svg	100
Grilled chicken dinner	1	130
Grilled chicken sandwich	1	435
Grilled chicken stir fried	1	865
Grilled salmon dinner	6 oz	210
Ham & Swiss sandwich	1	535
Hamburger, bacon & cheddar	1	875
Hamburger, big Texas BBQ	1	930
Hamburger, boca	1	615
Hamburger, classic	1	675
Hamburger, classic doubledecker	1	1375
Hamburger, classic w/ cheese	1	836
Hamburger, mushroom & Swiss	1	872
Hot fudge cake sundae	1 svg	620
Malted milk shake, chocolate	12 oz	585
Malted milk shake, vanilla	12 oz	585
Mashed potatoes	1 svg	105
Mashed potatoes w/ cheddar	1 svg	117
Mozzarella sticks, 8 per svg	1 svg	710
Onion rings	1 svg	380
Peaches and cream sundae	1	570
Pie, apple	1 slice	475
Pie, cherry	1 slice	630
Pie, chocolate peanut butter	1 slice	655
Pie, Hershey's chocolate chip	1 slice	600
Pie, Oreo cookies & cream	1 slice	650
Pot roast dinner	1	295
Roast turkey dinner	1	388
Reuben sandwich	1	580
Shake, chocolate	12 oz	560

RESTAURANT: (See other Foods and Beverages listed separately)	Serving Size	Calories
Shake, vanilla	12 oz	560
Shrimp scampi skillet dinner	1 svg	290
Sirloin steak dinner	8 oz	340
Slim slam	12 oz	495
Steak and shrimp dinner	9 oz	640
Super bird sandwich	1	· 620
T-bone steak dinner	14 oz	860
Two egg breakfast	1	825
Turkey breast sandwich	1	475
Vegetable rice pilaf	1 svg	85
Western wings roundup	20 oz	1515
Domino's Pizza	…	…
(1 slice= 1/8 pizza)	…	…
Medium 12-inch Pizzas	…	…
Cheese	…	…
Classic hand-tossed	1 slice	185
Crunchy thin crust	1 slice	135
Ultimate deep dish	1 slice	240
Beef	…	…
Classic hand-tossed	1 slice	225
Crunchy thin crust	1 slice	175
Ultimate deep dish	1 slice	277
Green pepper, mushroom, onion	…	…
Classic hand-tossed	1 slice	190
Crunchy thin crust	1 slice	142
Ultimate deep dish	1 slice	244
Ham	…	…
Classic hand-tossed	1 slice	195
Crunchy thin crust	1 slice	150
Ultimate deep dish	1 slice	250
Ham & pineapple	…	…
Classic hand-tossed	1 slice	200
Crunchy thin crust	1 slice	150
Ultimate deep dish	1 slice	250
Pepperoni	…	…
Classic hand-tossed	1 slice	223
Crunchy thin crust	1 slice	175
Ultimate deep dish	1 slice	275
Pepperoni & sausage	…	…
Classic hand-tossed	1 slice	255
Crunchy thin crust	1 slice	206
Ultimate deep dish	1 slice	307

RESTAURANT: (See other Foods and Beverages listed separately)	Serving Size	Calories
Sausage	...	...
Classic hand-tossed	1 slice	230
Crunchy thin crust	1 slice	181
Ultimate deep dish	1 slice	283
Large 14-inch Pizzas	...	...
Cheese	...	...
Classic hand-tossed	1 slice	256
Crunchy thin crust	1 slice	190
Ultimate deep dish	1 slice	336
Beef	...	...
Classic hand-tossed	1 slice	310
Crunchy thin crust	1 slice	243
Ultimate deep dish	1 slice	390
Green pepper, mushroom, onion	...	...
Classic hand-tossed	1 slice	263
Crunchy thin crust	1 slice	200
Ultimate deep dish	1 slice	343
Ham	...	...
Classic hand-tossed	1 slice	270
Crunchy thin crust	1 slice	204
Ultimate deep dish	1 slice	350
Ham & pineapple	...	...
Classic hand-tossed	1 slice	275
Crunchy thin crust	1 slice	207
Ultimate deep dish	1 slice	355
Pepperoni	...	...
Classic hand-tossed	1 slice	305
Crunchy thin crust	1 slice	237
Ultimate deep dish	1 slice	385
Pepperoni & sausage	...	...
Classic hand-tossed	1 slice	350
Crunchy thin crust	1 slice	282
Ultimate deep dish	1 slice	430
Sausage	...	...
Classic hand-tossed	1 slice	320
Crunchy thin crust	1 slice	250
Ultimate deep dish	1 slice	400
Side Orders & Condiments	...	...
Barbecue buffalo wings	1 piece	50
Blue cheese dipping sauce	1 svg	225
Bread sticks	1 piece	115
Buffalo chicken kickers	1 piece	47

RESTAURANT: (See other Foods and Beverages listed separately)	Serving Size	Calories
Cheesy bread	1 piece	125
Cinnamon stix	1 piece	125
Garlic sauce	1 svg	440
Hot buffalo wings	1 piece	45
Hot dipping sauce	1 svg	15
Marinara dipping sauce	1 svg	25
Ranch dipping sauce	1 svg	195
Sweet icing	1 svg	250
Dunkin' Donuts	...	...
Bagels	...	...
Berry berry	1	345
Blueberry	1	350
Cinnamon raisin	1	335
Everything	1	430
Garlic	1	410
Onion	1	375
Plain	1	360
Poppyseed	1	440
Salt	1	360
Sesame	1	455
Sourdough	1	340
Wheat	1	350
Cream cheese	...	...
Chive	2 oz	170
Garden vegetable	2 oz	170
Light	2 oz	110
Plain	2 oz	190
Salmon	2 oz	170
Shedd's buttermatch blend	1 Tbsp	80
Strawberry	2 oz	195
Cookies	...	...
Chocolate chunk	1	220
Chocolate chunk w/ walnuts	1	230
Oatmeal raisin pecan	1	220
White chocolate chunk	1	235
Danish	...	...
Apple	1	250
Cheese	1	275
Strawberry cheese	1	250
Donuts	...	...
Apple crumb	1	235
Apple & spice	1	200

RESTAURANT: (See other Foods and Beverages listed separately)	Serving Size	Calories
Bavarian kreme	1	210
Black raspberry	1	210
Blueberry cake	1	290
Blueberry crumb	1	240
Boston kreme	1	240
Chocolate coconut cake	1	300
Chocolate frosted cake	1	360
Chocolate frosted	1	200
Chocolate glazed cake	1	295
Chocolate kreme filled	1	270
Cinnamon cake	1	330
Double chocolate cake	1	310
French cruller	1	150
Glazed cake	1	350
Glazed	1	180
Jelly filled	1	210
Maple frosted	1	210
Marble frosted	1	200
Old fashioned cake	1	300
Powdered cake	1	330
Strawberry	1	210
Strawberry frosted	1	210
Sugar raised	1	170
Vanilla kreme filled	1	170
Whole white glazed cake	1	310
Donut-Fancies	...	...
Apple fritter	1	300
Bow tie donut	1	300
Chocolate frosted coffee roll	1	290
Chocolate iced Bismarck	1	340
Coffee roll	1	270
Éclair	1	270
Glazed fritter	1	260
Maple frosted coffee roll	1	290
Vanilla frosted coffee roll	1	290
Donut-Munchkins	...	...
Cinnamon cake	4	275
Glazed	5	200
Glazed cake	3	280
Glazed chocolate cake	3	200
Jelly filled	5	210
Lemon filled	4	170

RESTAURANT: (See other Foods and Beverages listed separately)	Serving Size	Calories
Plain cake	4	270
Powdered cake	4	270
Sugar raised	7	220
Donut-Sticks	…	…
Cinnamon cake	1	450
Glazed cake	1	490
Glazed chocolate cake	1	470
Jelly	1	530
Plain cake	1	420
Powdered cake	1	450
Muffins	…	…
Banana walnut	1	545
Blueberry	1	490
Carrot walnut spice	1	600
Chocolate chip	1	590
Coffee cake with topping	1	710
Corn	1	510
Cranberry orange	1	460
Honey bran raisin	1	490
Reduced fat blueberry	1	450
Other Misc. Items	…	…
Apple pie	1 svg	615
Apple pie a la mode	1 svg	810
Biscuit, plain	1	250
Croissant, plain	1	330
Scone, maple walnut	1	470
Scone, raspberry white choc.	1	450
Sandwiches, Breakfast type	…	…
Bagel w/ egg, bacon, cheese	1	500
Bagel w/ egg, ham, cheese	1	500
Bagel w/ egg, sausage, cheese	1	675
Biscuit w/ egg & cheese	1	360
Biscuit w/ sausage, egg, cheese	1	560
Croissant w/ egg, ham, cheese	1	470
English muffin w/egg, cheese	1	270
English muffin w/ egg, bacon & cheese	1	310
English muffin w/ egg, ham, & cheese	1	310
Beverages	…	…
Cappuccino	10 oz	80
Cappuccino with sugar	10 oz	130

84

RESTAURANT: (See other Foods and Beverages listed separately)	Serving Size	Calories
Coffee	10 oz	15
Coffee with cream	10 oz	70
Coffee with cream and sugar	10 oz	120
Coffee with milk	10 oz	35
Coffee with milk and sugar	10 oz	80
Coffee with skim milk	10 oz	25
Coffee w/ skim milk & sugar	10 oz	70
Coffee with sugar	10 oz	60
Coffee coolatta with 2% milk	16 oz	190
Coffee coolatta with cream	16 oz	350
Coffee coolatta with milk	16 oz	210
Coffee coolatta w/skim milk	16 oz	170
Coolatta, strawberry fruit	16 oz	290
Coolatta, vanilla bean	16 oz	440
Dunkaccino	10 oz	230
Espresso	2 oz	1
Espresso with sugar	2 oz	30
Hot chocolate	10 oz	220
Latte, plain	10 oz	120
Latte with sugar	10 oz	160
Latte w/ Caramel swirl	10 oz	230
Latte w/ Mocha swirl	10 oz	230
Iced coffee	16 oz	15
Iced coffee with cream	16 oz	70
Iced coffee w/cream & sugar	16 oz	120
Iced coffee with milk	16 oz	35
Iced coffee w/ milk and sugar	16 oz	80
Iced coffee with skim milk	16 oz	25
Iced coffee w/skim milk, sugar	16 oz	70
Iced latte	16 oz	120
Iced latte with sugar	16 oz	170
Iced caramel swirl latte	16 oz	240
Iced mocha swirl latte	16 oz	240
Vanilla chai	10 oz	230
Tea, plain, w/o milk or sugar	…	…
Decaffeinated tea	10 oz	0
Earl Grey tea	10 oz	0
English breakfast tea	10 oz	0
Green tea	10 oz	0
Regular tea	10 oz	0
Regular tea w/ lemon	10 oz	0
Tea w/ regular milk, no sugar	10 oz	25

RESTAURANT: (See other Foods and Beverages listed separately)	Serving Size	Calories
Tea w/ regular milk and sugar	10 oz	70
Tea w/ skim milk, no sugar	10 oz	25
Tea w/ skim milk and sugar	10 oz	60
Hardees	…	…
Apple cinnamon raisin biscuit	1	200
Bacon & egg biscuit	1	575
Bacon, egg & cheese biscuit	1	610
Baked beans	1 svg	170
Big chocolate chip cookie	1	280
Big country bacon	1 svg	820
Big country sausage	1 svg	995
Big roast beef	1	465
Biscuits w/ gravy	1 svg	495
Cheeseburger	1	310
Chicken, breast	1 piece	370
Chicken, leg	1 piece	170
Chicken, thigh	1 piece	330
Chicken, wing	1 piece	195
Chicken fillet sandwich	1	480
Chocolate cone	1	180
Chocolate shake	1	375
Cole slaw	1 svg	240
Cool twist cone	1	180
Country ham biscuit	1	430
Cravin bacon cheeseburger	1	690
Fat free French dressing	1 svg	70
Fisherman's fillet	1	565
French fries, large	1	430
French fries, medium	1	350
French fries, small	1	240
Frisco ham sandwich	1	500
Frisco sandwich	1	720
Garden salad	1	220
Gravy, 1.5 oz	1 svg	22
Grilled chicken	1	350
Chilled chicken salad	1	150
Ham biscuit	1	400
Ham, egg, & cheese biscuit	1	540
Hamburger	1	270
Hot fudge sundae	1	180
Hot ham & cheese	1	310
Jelly biscuit	1	440

RESTAURANT: (See other Foods and Beverages listed separately)	Serving Size	Calories
Mashed potatoes	1 svg	70
Mesquite bacon cheeseburger	1	370
Mushroom & Swiss burger	1	490
Pancakes, 3 per svg	1 svg	280
Peach cobbler	1 svg	310
Peach shake	1	390
Quarter Lb double cheeseburger	1	470
Ranch dressing	1 svg	290
Regular hash rounds	1 svg	230
Regular roast beef	1	320
Rise & shine biscuit	1	390
Sausage biscuit	1	510
Sausage & egg biscuit	1	630
Side salad, w/o dressing	1	25
Strawberry shake	1	420
Strawberry sundae	1	210
The boss	1	570
The works burger	1	530
Thousand island dressing	1 svg	250
Ultimate omelet biscuit	1	570
Vanilla cone	1	170
Vanilla shake	1	350
Jack-In-The-Box	…	…
Breakfast Jack	1	295
Breakfast sandwich, sourdough	1	380
Carrot cake	1 piece	365
Cheeseburger, regular	1	320
Cheeseburger, double	1	450
Cheeseburger, ultimate	1	1025
Cheesecake	1 piece	310
Chicken pita fajita	1	290
Chicken sandwich, regular	1	400
Chicken sandwich, Caesar	1	520
Chicken sandwich, grilled	1	430
Chicken sandwich, spicy	1	560
Chicken sandwich, super	1	615
Chicken strips, 6 per svg	1 svg	450
Chicken teriyaki	1 svg	580
Egg roll	1 piece	150
Egg rolls, 5 piece serving	5 piece	745
French fries, curly	1	360
French fries, jumbo size	1	400

RESTAURANT: (See other Foods and Beverages listed separately)	Serving Size	Calories
French fries, regular size	1	350
French fries, small	1	220
French fries, super size	1	590
Hamburger	1	280
Hash browns	2 oz	160
Jalapenos, stuffed	1 svg	600
Jumbo Jack	1	560
Jumbo Jack w/ cheese	1	650
Onion rings	1 svg	380
Pancake platter	1 svg	400
Potato wedges, bacon & cheddar	1 svg	795
Sausage croissant	1	675
Scrambled egg pocket	1	430
Shake, cappuccino	1 large	625
Shake, chocolate	1 large	625
Shake, strawberry	1 large	630
Shake, vanilla	1 large	615
Supreme croissant	1	570
Taco	1	185
Taco monster	1	285
Kentucky Fried Chicken	...	...
Barbecue baked beans	1 svg	185
Biscuit	1	180
Breast, extra tasty crispy	1	470
Breast, hot & spicy	1	520
Breast, original recipe	1	400
Breast, tender roast	1	255
Chunky chicken pot pie	1	775
Coleslaw	5 oz	180
Cornbread	1 piece	228
Corn on the cob	1	190
Crispy strips, 3 pieces/svg	1 svg	260
Drumstick, original recipe	1	160
Drumstick, tender roast	1	100
Green beans	1 svg	45
Hot wings, 6 pieces/svg	1 svg	470
Kentucky nuggets , 6 pieces/svg	1 svg	285
Macaroni and cheese	med	180
Original recipe chicken sandwich	... 1	... 495
Potato salad	1 svg	230
Potato wedges	1 svg	280

RESTAURANT: (See other Foods and Beverages listed separately)	Serving Size	Calories
Potatoes, mashed	1 svg	120
Red beans and rice	1 svg	130
Thigh, extra tasty crispy or hot	1	370
Thigh, original recipe	1	255
Thigh, tender roast	1	205
Value BBQ chicken sandwich	1	255
Wing, extra tasty crispy or hot	1	210
Wing, original recipe	1	140
Wing, tender roast	1	121
Krispy Kreme Doughnuts	…	…
Apple fritter	1	385
Caramel creme crunch	1	350
Chocolate iced cake	1	270
Chocolate iced cake w/ sprinkles	1	290
Chocolate iced crème filled	1	350
Chocolate iced cruller	1	290
Chocolate iced custard filled	1	300
Chocolate iced glazed	1	250
Chocolate iced glazed, sprinkles	1	200
Chocolate malted kreme	1	395
Cinnamon apple filled	1	290
Cinnamon bun	1	260
Cinnamon sugar cake	1	280
Cinnamon twist	1	230
Coffee & kreme	1	360
Dulce de leche	1	295
Glazed blueberry cake	1	340
Glazed blueberry filled	1	290
Glazed cinnamon	1	210
Glazed crème filled	1	345
Glazed cruller	1	240
Glazed custard filled	1	290
Glazed devil's food cake	1	340
Glazed lemon filled	1	290
Glazed sour cream	1	340
Glazed raspberry filled	1	300
Glazed strawberry filled	1	290
Glazed twist	1	210
Honey and oat	1	340
Key lime pie	1	330
Maple iced	1	240
Maple iced cake	1	270

RESTAURANT: (See other Foods and Beverages listed separately)	Serving Size	Calories
New York cheesecake	1	330
Original glazed	1	200
Powdered blueberry filled	1	290
Powdered cake	1	280
Powdered crème filled	1	345
Powdered raspberry	1	300
Powdered strawberry filled	1	260
Pumpkin spice cake	1	340
Sugar coated	1	200
Traditional cake	1	230
Vanilla iced cake w/ sprinkles	1	270
Vanilla iced crème filled	1	345
Vanilla iced custard filled	1	290
Vanilla iced glazed	1	240
Vanilla iced raspberry filled	1	355
Vanilla iced raspberry glazed	1	355
Long John Silver's	...	...
Cheesesticks, 3 per svg	1 svg	165
Chicken, battered plank	1	145
Chicken sandwich	1	340
Chicken sandwich w/ cheese	1	390
Clam chowder	1 svg	525
Clams, breaded	1 svg	250
Cole slaw	4 oz	170
Crabcake	1	150
Fish, battered	1 piece	230
Fish, battered, junior size	1 piece	120
Fish, country breaded	1 piece	200
Fish w/lemon crumb	2 piece	240
Fish sandwich	1	430
Fish sandwich w/ cheese	1	485
Fish sandwich, ultimate	1	490
French fries, regular size	1	250
French fries, large size	1	420
Grilled chicken salad	1	140
Hushpuppies	2 piece	120
Ocean chef salad	1	128
Pie, banana split sundae	1 svg	300
Pie, chocolate crème	1 svg	285
Pie, Dutch apple	1 svg	290
Pie, pecan	1 svg	390
Pie, strawberries & cream	1 svg	280

RESTAURANT: (See other Foods and Beverages listed separately)	Serving Size	Calories
Pineapple crème cheesecake	1 svg	310
Shrimp, battered	1 piece	45
Shrimp, battered, popcorn	1 svg	325
McDonald's	...	...
Apple bran muffin, lowfat	1	300
Apple Danish	1	360
Apple pie, baked	1	260
Arch deluxe	1	550
Arch deluxe with bacon	1	590
Bacon, egg & cheese biscuit	1	440
Barbecue sauce	1 svg	45
Big mac	1	560
Biscuit, plain	1	260
Breakfast burrito	1	320
Caesar salad	1	160
Chef salad	1	230
Cheese Danish	1	410
Cheeseburger	1	320
Chicken McNuggets, 4 pieces	1 svg	190
Chicken McNuggets, 6 pieces	1 svg	290
Chicken McNuggets, 9 pieces	1 svg	430
Chocolate chip cookie	1	170
Chocolate shake, small	1	360
Cinnamon roll	1	400
Crispy chicken deluxe	1	500
Croutons	1 svg	50
Egg McMuffin	1	290
English muffin	1	140
Fat free herb vinegar dressing	1 svg	50
Fish fillet sandwich	1	560
French fries, large	1	450
French fries, small	1	210
Garden salad	1	35
Grilled chicken deluxe	1	440
Grilled chicken salad deluxe	1	120
Hamburger	1	260
Hash browns	1 svg	130
Honey dressing	1 svg	45
Honey mustard dressing	1 svg	50
Hot caramel sundae	1	360
Hot fudge sundae	1	340
Hot mustard	1 svg	60

RESTAURANT: (See other Foods and Beverages listed separately)	Serving Size	Calories
Hotcakes, plain	1 svg	310
Hotcakes w/ syrup & margarine	1 svg	580
Mayonnaise, light	1 svg	40
McDonaldland cookie	1	180
Quarter pounder	1	420
Quarter pounder with cheese	1	530
Red French reduced cal dressing	1 svg	160
Sausage (w/o biscuit)	1 svg	170
Sausage biscuit w/ egg	1	505
Sausage McMuffin	1	360
Sausage McMuffin with egg	1	440
Scrambled eggs, 2 per svg	1 svg	160
Strawberry shake, small	1	360
Strawberry sundae	1	290
Sweet & sour sauce	1 svg	50
Vanilla cone, reduced fat	1	150
Vanilla shake, small	1	360
Panda Express Chinese Food	…	…
Beef dishes	…	…
Beef with broccoli	6 oz	150
Beef with string beans	6 oz	170
Chicken dishes	…	…
Black pepper chicken	6 oz	180
Chicken & orange sauce	6 oz	480
Chicken with mushrooms	6 oz	130
Chicken with string beans	6 oz	170
Hot spicy chicken w/ peanuts	6 oz	200
Mandarin chicken	6 oz	250
Potatoes with chicken	6 oz	220
Sweet & sour chicken	4 oz	310
Pork dishes	…	…
Barbecue pork	5 oz	350
Sweet & sour pork	4 oz	410
Vegetable dishes	…	…
Mixed vegetables	6 oz	70
String beans w/fried tofu	6 oz	180
Vegetable chow mein	8 oz	330
Rice	…	…
Fried rice w/vegetables	8 oz	390
Steamed rice	8 oz	330
Appetizers	…	…
Fried shrimp	6 piece	260

RESTAURANT: (See other Foods and Beverages listed separately)	Serving Size	Calories
Chicken egg roll	1	190
Vegetable spring roll	1	80
Sauces	…	…
Hot mustard sauce	1 svg	18
Hot sauce	2 tsp	10
Mandarin sauce	2 oz	70
Sweet & sour sauce	2 oz	60
Soy sauce	1 Tbsp	16
Papa John's Pizza	…	…
Original crust pizza, large-14"	…	…
Cheese	1 slice	290
Pepperoni	1 slice	345
Sausage	1 slice	335
Sausage, pepperoni & beef	1 slice	405
Sausage & pepperoni	1 slice	348
Vegetable garden fresh pizza	1 slice	287
Works, the works pizza	1 slice	370
Specialty pizzas	…	…
Alfredo, spinach	1 slice	303
Alfredo, vegetable & chicken	1 slice	310
Chicken and bacon BBQ	1 slice	370
Hawaiian BBQ chicken	1 slice	375
Thin crust pizza, large-14"	…	…
Cheese	1 slice	240
Pepperoni	1 slice	295
Sausage	1 slice	303
Sausage, pepperoni & beef	1 slice	371
Sausage & pepperoni	1 slice	298
Vegetable garden fresh pizza	1 slice	228
Works, the works pizza	1 slice	315
Specialty pizzas	…	…
Alfredo, spinach	1 slice	251
Alfredo, vegetable & chicken	1 slice	276
Chicken and bacon BBQ	1 slice	336
Hawaiian BBQ chicken	1 slice	324
Side items	…	…
BBQ dipping sauce	1 svg	48
Bread sticks	1 svg	140
Buffalo hot sauce	1 svg	25
Cheese sauce	1 svg	60
Cheese sticks	1 svg	180
Chicken strips	1 svg	83

RESTAURANT: (See other Foods and Beverages listed separately)	Serving Size	Calories
Cinnapie	1 svg	114
Garlic sauce	1 svg	235
Honey mustard dipping sauce	1 svg	190
Pizza sauce	1 svg	25
Ranch dipping sauce	1 svg	140
Pizza Hut	...	...
Bread stick	1	130
Bread stick sauce for dipping	1 svg	30
Buffalo wings	4	200
Cavatini pasta	1 svg	485
Cavatini pasta supreme	1 svg	565
Cherry dessert pizza	1 slice	250
Garlic bread	1 slice	150
Ham and cheese sandwich	1	555
Hand tossed pizza	...	...
Beef	1 slice	260
Cheese	1 slice	235
Ham	1 slice	215
Pepperoni	1 slice	238
Sausage	1 slice	265
Supreme	1 slice	284
Pan pizza	...	...
Beef	1 slice	285
Cheese	1 slice	260
Ham	1 slice	240
Pepperoni	1 slice	265
Supreme	1 slice	310
Veggie	1 slice	245
Spaghetti with marina sauce	1 svg	490
Spaghetti with meat sauce	1 svg	600
Spaghetti with meatballs	1 svg	850
Stuffed crust pizza	...	...
Beef	1 slice	465
Cheese	1 slice	445
Ham	1 slice	404
Pepperoni	1 slice	440
Sausage	1 slice	480
Supreme sandwich	1	640
Thin & crispy pizza	...	...
Beef	1 slice	230
Cheese	1 slice	205
Pepperoni	1 slice	215

RESTAURANT: (See other Foods and Beverages listed separately)	Serving Size	Calories
Sausage	1 slice	235
Supreme	1 slice	255
Veggie	1 slice	185
Subway	…	…
Six Inch subs	…	…
BLT on wheat	1	325
BLT on white	1	310
Classic Italian BMT wheat	1	460
Classic Italian BMT white	1	445
Cold cut trio on wheat	1	380
Cold cut trio on white	1	360
Ham on wheat	1	300
Ham on white	1	287
Meatball on wheat	1	420
Meatball on white	1	405
Pizza sub wheat	1	465
Pizza sub white	1	448
Roast beef on wheat	1	305
Roast beef on white	1	288
Roasted chicken breast, wheat	1	348
Roasted chicken breast, white	1	332
Spicy Italian wheat	1	482
Spice Italian white	1	465
Steak & cheese wheat	1	395
Steak & cheese white	1	383
Subway club wheat	1	310
Subway club white	1	295
Subway melt wheat	1	382
Subway melt white	1	366
Subway seafood & crab, wheat	1	430
Subway seafood & crab, white	1	415
Tuna on wheat	1	542
Tuna on white	1	527
Turkey breast & ham, wheat	1	280
Turkey breast & ham, white	1	295
Turkey on wheat	1	289
Turkey on white	1	273
Veggie delite wheat	1	235
Veggie delite white	1	220
Taco subs	…	…
Chicken taco sub wheat	1	436
Chicken taco sub white	1	421

RESTAURANT: (See other Foods and Beverages listed separately)	Serving Size	Calories
Beverages	…	…
Berry lishus drink	small	113
Peach pizazz drink	small	103
Pineapple delight drink	small	133
Sunrise refresher drink	small	119
Cookies	…	…
Brazil nut & chocolate chip	1	230
Chocolate chip cookie	1	210
Chocolate chip, M&M cookie	1	210
Chocolate chunk cookie	1	210
Oatmeal raisin cookie	1	205
Peanut butter cookie	1	220
Sugar cookie	1	230
White chip macadamia nut	1	235
Taco Bell	…	…
Bacon cheeseburger	1	565
Bean burrito	1	378
Big beef meximelt	1	300
Big beef nachos supreme	1	435
Big beef supreme	1	518
Breakfast cheese quesadilla	1	390
Breakfast quesadilla with bacon	1	465
Breakfast quesadilla w/ sausage	1	440
Burrito supreme	1	440
Cheddar cheese	1 svg	30
Cheese quesadilla	1	370
Chicken club	1	540
Chicken fajita	1	460
Chicken fajita supreme	1	500
Chicken quesadilla	1	420
Chili with cheese	1 svg	330
Cinnamon twists	1 svg	140
Country burrito	1	270
Double bacon & egg burrito	1	480
Double decker supreme	1	390
Double decker taco	1	340
Fiesta burrito	1	280
Grande burrito	1	420
Green sauce	1 svg	5
Guacamole	1 svg	35
Hot taco sauce	1 svg	1
Kid's soft taco roll-up	1	290

RESTAURANT: (See other Foods and Beverages listed separately)	Serving Size	Calories
Light chicken	1	310
Light chicken soft taco	1	180
Light chicken supreme	1	430
Light kid's chicken soft taco	1	180
Mexican pizza	1	570
Mexican rice	1 svg	190
Mild taco sauce	1 svg	1
Nacho cheese sauce	1 svg	120
Nachos	1	315
Nachos belle grande	1	740
Pepper jack cheese	1 svg	25
Picante sauce	1 svg	1
Pinto & cheese	1	195
Red sauce	1 svg	10
Salsa	1 svg	25
Seven layer burrito	1	540
Soft taco	1	210
Soft taco, BLT	1	340
Soft taco, steak	1	510
Steak fajita	1	465
Taco, hard shell	1	200
Taco salad	1	170
Taco salad with salsa w/o shell	1	420
Taco supreme	1	260
Tostada	1	305
Veggie fajita	1	420
Veggie fajita supreme	1	465
Wendy's	...	...
Baked potato w/ bacon & cheese	1	535
Baked potato w/ broccoli, cheese	1	470
Baked potato with cheese	1	570
Baked potato w/ chili & cheese	1	625
Baked potato, sour cream, chive	1	370
Big bacon classic hamburger	1	640
Breaded chicken sandwich	1	450
Caesar salad	1	110
Cheeseburger kids' meal	1	310
Chicken Caesar pita	1	485
Chicken club sandwich	1	520
Chicken nuggets, 5 per svg	1 svg	190
Chili (large)	1 svg	310
Chili (small)	1 svg	210

RESTAURANT: (See other Foods and Beverages listed separately)	Serving Size	Calories
Chocolate chip cookie	1	270
Classic Greek pita	1	440
Classic hamburger, single	1	360
Classic hamburger w/ everything	1	420
Coleslaw	1 svg	45
French fries (biggie)	1	470
French fries (small)	1	270
French fries (super)	1	570
Frosty (large)	1	570
Frosty (medium)	1	460
Frosty (small)	1	340
Garden ranch chicken pita	1	480
Garden veggie pita	1	400
Grilled chicken fillet, w/o bun	1	100
Grilled chicken salad	1	190
Grilled chicken sandwich	1	290
Hamburger kids' meal	1	270
Junior bacon cheeseburger	1	445
Junior cheeseburger	1	320
Junior cheeseburger deluxe	1	360
Junior hamburger	1	270
Kaiser bun	1	190
Sandwich bun	1	160
Spicy chicken sandwich	1	415
Strawberry banana dessert	1	30
Taco salad	1	375
White Castle	....	...
Breakfast sandwich, regular	1	335
Cheeseburger	1	235
Cheeseburger with bacon	1	200
Cheeseburger, double	1	285
Cheesesticks, 5 per svg	1 svg	490
Chicken rings, 6 per svg	1 svg	310
Chicken ring sandwich	1	170
Chocolate shake	14 oz	220
Fish sandwich	1	160
French fries, small	1	115
Hamburger	1	135
Hamburger, double	1	235
Onion rings, 8 per svg	1 svg	455
Vanilla shake	14 oz	228

EASY LIFETIME
DIET & EXERCISE GUIDE

It is possible to take total control of your weight. The facts, tips, and ideas in this guide provide the "need to know" essentials of calories, exercise, and weight management. This guide along with the calorie counter gives the power and the knowledge for permanent solutions to weight management, while promoting good overall health.

This plan is safe, effective, easy to follow, and fits into any lifestyle. Learn the secrets to weight management, and simple exercise routines that lead to a lifetime of health, well being, and total success in weight control.

Fad diets, crash diets, and starvation diets are not recommended. Any temporary weight loss on a crash diet, will return quickly once normal eating habits are resumed. There are also potential adverse health effects from any type of quick weight loss diet, and data shows that starvation diets also lead to a slower metabolism.

For total lifetime weight management, it is better to have a diet plan that is fairly easy to maintain on a permanent basis; one that hardly feels like a diet at all.

This diet plan is very simple: First choose your ideal body weight. You may know exactly what is right for you, or you can refer to the "Ideal Body Weight" chart. You then calculate the number of daily calories needed to achieve that weight. (Calculations discussed later). You can eat satisfying and well-balanced variety of foods, including all your favorite foods, while making better food choices by counting calories. Read over the Healthy Diet Basics, and the Easy Weight Loss Secrets. If you want to achieve optimal health, you should add a simple exercise routine to your day. Exercise also helps speed up weight loss, and makes lifetime weight management much easier.

When trying to lose weight, several factors come into play that affect the speed of weight loss. This includes:

- How many pounds you are above your ideal weight. Generally, the more you weigh, the faster you will lose weight. Losing and keeping off the last 10 pounds is usually the most difficult. Losing 5 to 7 pounds per month is a healthy goal.
- Your commitment to counting and cutting calories; and your commitment to get active with exercise.
- Your metabolism. As you age, metabolism naturally slows down. Exercise speeds up the metabolism. Heredity is also a factor; some people have a faster metabolism than others.

Healthy Diet Basics

The following is a list of important facts, and healthy tips to keep in mind for smart weight management. These tips will help in achieving and maintaining your ideal weight.

Drink 6 to 8 glasses of water every day. Water helps to cleanse and purify the body, and improves overall health.

Take a multi-vitamin and mineral supplement every day. This helps to assure that you are obtaining all the essential nutrients your body needs.

Eat a variety of foods every day from all of the food groups. Variety and balance in the food groups helps to assure proper nutrition and good health. All types of foods contain varying amounts of vitamins, minerals, and nutrients. The food groups are:

- Bread, grains, oats, wheat, cereal, rice, and pasta.
  (Good source of carbs and fiber, some protein).

- Fruits and vegetables.
  (Fruits and vegetables contain many
    nutrients, fiber, and antioxidants).

- Dairy products including milk, and cheese.
  (High in protein and carbs, some are high in fat).

- Meat products including beef, pork, chicken, fish, and eggs.
  (High in protein, some are high in fat).

- Fats, oils, and sweets. Minimize intake of this food group.
  (Very high in fat and/or sugar).

The USDA recommendations for variety and balance in daily caloric intake follows:

- 50% to 60% from carbohydrates
- 12% to 20% from proteins
- Less than 30% from fats

For example, in an 1800 calorie diet, for a 120 pound adult, the USDA recommends the following daily intake for optimal nutritional health:

Carbohydrates: 250 grams
                (about 55% of total caloric intake)

Protein: 54 grams
            (about 16% of total caloric intake)

Fat: Less than 58 grams
       (less than 30% of total caloric intake)

Fiber: 23 grams or more. Fiber is found in carbohydrates and supplies multiple health benefits. Fiber is especially good for the heart and colon. Some studies indicate that an increase in fiber with the proper balance of protein increases the metabolism naturally, resulting in faster weight loss, and easier weight management.

Carbohydrates can be classified as simple, such as sugar, or complex. The complex carbohydrates are healthy and contain many nutrients.

Carbohydrates also include fiber. Foods high in complex carbs, such as bread and rice contain many vitamins and minerals. Carbs also contain starch and sugar. Sugar is the so-called "bad carb"; high in calories with little nutritional value. You can usually identify a bad carb because it is sweet.

Some diets promote higher intake of protein, with lower intake of carbohydrates. This does promote faster weight loss in many people, however, nutrition experts agree that a well balanced diet with higher intake of carbohydrates, less protein, and less fat is safer and healthier. A minor increase in protein intake, with a minor decrease in carbohydrate intake is a better option if considering a high protein/low carb diet. The extremes of almost all protein and fat, with almost no carbohydrate intake can have serious health consequences. Many high protein foods are also high in fat and cholesterol, and some are high in sodium (processed meats). Health problems noted in high protein, high fat, low carb diets include: kidney failure, increased risk of heart disease due to increased cholesterol levels, and increased risk of cancer.

All About Calories & Weight

Simply put, if you eat fewer calories, you will lose weight. There are 3500 calories in one pound. For every 3500 calories you cut out of your diet, you will lose one pound of body weight. Calories provide energy. You need calories and the energy derived from calories to live. However, if you consume more calories than your body needs, the result is weight gain. For the safest, healthiest weight loss, you need to maintain the proper caloric intake, balance your food groups, and increase your physical activity level. This leads to good health, good nutrition, and easy to maintain, long lasting results.

You can choose your perfect weight for yourself, or refer to the ideal body weight chart. Then you just determine the number of calories you need per day to achieve that weight. For example: Let's say your ideal weight is 120 pounds, and you have a moderately active lifestyle. You need approximately 1800 calories per day. (See the lifestyle activity levels and factors). 1800 calories per day is a satisfying amount of food in most people's opinion. 1800 calories per day leaves plenty of room for good variety, balance, and nutrition. You just need to learn to make smart food choices, and counting calories is the best way.

Read over the calorie counter. Get to know which foods are naturally lower in calories. Reducing your caloric intake, and managing your weight is so much easier once you learn which types of foods are high in calories, and which types of foods are low in calories.

Calorie counting gets easier over time, and after a while it is like second nature. After a few months of using a calorie counter, most people have memorized the approximate calorie counts of favorite foods. While it is true every calorie counts in weight management, it is also true that every bit of activity also counts. It is almost impossible to measure exactly how many calories you burn in a day; you would have to measure calorie expenditure every time you stand up, even every time you move. It is, however, easy to figure approximately how many calories you need, and how many you burn per day with the simple formulas in this book. So, you do not need to spend lots of time counting every calorie. Instead, try rounding and averaging calories to save time, but don't cheat yourself by neglecting to count the majority of your calories.

After some practice counting calories, you won't even need to write down the daily calorie counts. Many experienced calorie counting people are able to keep a daily running total in the back of their mind.

How many calories do you need per day?

There are complicated formulas and expensive tests to determine your caloric requirements based on basal metabolism. A very simple rule of thumb is to choose your ideal weight and multiply by 15 to determine your daily caloric requirements. This formula is correct for moderately active, healthy adults over age 18. The activity levels and factors are discussed in the next section.

If you are extremely active, your caloric requirements will be higher. If you are sedentary, your caloric requirements will be lower.

Caloric requirements decrease with age as the metabolism slows down. Every 5-10 years, you will likely notice a few pounds creeping on despite your best efforts. You will need to consume slightly less calories and/or exercise a little more to stay at the same weight. Note: Caloric requirements can be significantly increased during any illness. Caloric requirements can be reduced in cases of hypothyroidism.

Formula for Calculating Daily Calories Needed:

Multiply your ideal body weight by your activity factor to determine daily caloric requirements.

Example: A moderately active adult who wants to weigh 120 pounds, needs 1800 calories per day.

$$120 \times 15 = 1800$$

Lifestyle Activity Levels & Factors

Sedentary Lifestyle   (Factor = 12)
Sitting most of the day, no formal exercise program.

Moderately Active Lifestyle   (Factor = 15)
Performs regular moderately strenuous exercise program at least 3 times per week for at least 20 minutes per session. Good amount of walking and activity in normal daily routine.

Vigorously Active Lifestyle   (Factor = 18)

Extremely active. Performs regular strenuous exercise at least 5 times per week for at least 30 minutes per session. Exercise program includes running or jogging at fast pace, high impact aerobic type exercise, or equally strenuous exercise. Daily routine and/or job include lots of physical activity.

If you fall somewhere in the middle, your activity factor will fall somewhere in the middle of these activity factors.

Calorie expenditure describes the process of the body utilizing or burning calories for energy. Different activities burn calories at different levels. You can measure your overall lifestyle activity level and the factors by using this chart. You can then make adjustments to your activity level, and add exercises that help burn calories faster.

Tip: Every time you perform a physical activity or exercise, you are burning more calories than if you are sitting. So a key to losing weight faster, is to GET ACTIVE! Take the stairs whenever possible, take a walk after eating, find an exercise or activity you enjoy, and add it to your daily routine. Adding a simple exercise like walking, biking, or swimming to your daily routine, for 20 minutes per day, 3 to 5 days per week will help to speed up weight loss, increase muscle tone, and increase your energy level.

Note: As you age your metabolism naturally slows down. Even expert lifelong diet and exercise enthusiasts report that around age 30 to 40 they have to eat a little less or exercise a little more to maintain the same weight; and they report that about every 5 to 10 years as the metabolism slows down, they need to adjust their diet and exercise plan slightly in order to maintain the same weight.

Which exercises burn more calories?

Simply, the more strenuous the exercise, the more calories you burn. You can also gauge how vigorous the exercise is by checking your heart rate. (This is discussed later.)

Weight training/weightlifting is a little different than other exercises. You may or may not increase you heart rate as much as with other exercises, but you are still doing yourself a world of good. Weight training is very effective at toning muscles and increasing lean muscle mass. This means you will have less fat and more muscle on your body. Muscle also weighs more than fat, so you will need more calories per day to maintain your weight. You can also achieve your ideal physique by adjusting the amount of weights you train with, and the number of repetitions you perform. You can choose to be anywhere from lean and well-toned to very muscular. To achieve that, women can use light weights and more repetitions. Men can use heavier weights with less repetitions.

An exercise is classified as aerobic if you can achieve and maintain your maximum heart rate range for at least 20 minutes, and preferably 30 minutes. Aerobic exercise provides a multitude of health benefits:

- Increased energy levels
- Faster weight loss
- Improved overall health
- Lower blood pressure and lower resting heart rate (This is a long-term beneficial aspect of aerobic exercise).

Before beginning an exercise, check your normal resting heart rate. The normal for an adult is 60 to 100 beats per minute, with 80 being the average normal value. Count the heartbeat for 15 seconds and multiply by 4 to calculate beats per minute. Then check your heart rate periodically while performing an exercise, to be sure you are maintaining the aerobic level.

Using heart rate to calculate aerobic exercise level:

Your target heart rate while exercising is calculated as follows:

220 (minus your age) x (75%)

Example: for a 35-year-old:
220 – 35 = 185 x 75% = 139

In this example, the 35-year-old can gauge the exercise activity level by the heart rate increase from a resting heart rate of 80 to the aerobic exercise heart rate of 139. The heart rate should be checked periodically to gauge the aerobic level.

Note: If your heart rate is much higher than calculated in the formula, you should stop exercising, and consult your physician before restarting aerobic exercise. Also, any illness including a fever can increase heart rate, so the heart rates given here are for normal healthy adults only. Always check with your doctor before beginning any exercise program.

Calorie expenditure increases with more strenuous exercise and activity. This chart reveals some common activities and the number of calories burned per hour during these activities.

Calorie expenditure chart*

Activity/Exercise	*Calories burned per hour	
	Female	**Male**
Sitting quietly	**60**	**80**
Standing still	**75**	**100**

Light activity/exercise
  Cleaning the house
  Walking slowly/strolling
  Playing golf
  Light weight training/weightlifting
	210	**250**

Moderate activity/exercise
  Bicycling at 6 mph
  Fast power walking at 3.5 mph
  Swimming at a moderate pace
  Low/Moderate impact aerobics
  Dancing at moderate pace
  Moderate weight training/weightlifting
  Playing basketball or tennis
	330	**410**

Strenuous activity/exercise
  High impact aerobics
  Swimming very fast
  Jogging/running at 8 mph or faster
  Jumping rope very fast
  Stair stepping
  Cross country skiing
	620	**800**

*Calories burned per hour in this example are approximate values for a normal healthy adult female weighing 130 pounds, or a normal, healthy adult male weighing 165 pounds.

Activity / Exercise Tips

Choose an activity you enjoy, and perform it regularly for at least 20 minutes per day, at least three days per week. This will promote faster weight loss, easier weight management, improved overall health, and improved sense of well being.

This exercise can be as simple as walking. You can walk outside, or use a treadmill, or simulate a walk inside while watching your favorite television program, or catching up on the news. You should walk at a fast pace, but one that is comfortable to you. Don't walk so fast that you get short of breath. Your stamina and endurance will increase the longer you continue. If you are walking inside, be sure to really lift your feet off the floor. As you walk, be sure to swing your arms back and forth.

Other simple methods include bicycling outdoors or on an indoor stationary bike. Also try performing aerobics with an exercise video, kickboxing video, or dance video, in endless varieties of styles and speeds. Choose light aerobics first and work your way up to high impact aerobics when that feels comfortable.

If you want to tone up your muscles faster, and burn lots of extra calories, you can hold weights in your hands while you exercise. You can also try strapping weights on your wrists and ankles while you are exercising, while working around the house, taking a walk, or riding a stationary bike. Start with low weights like one pound weights for the arms and two or three pound weights for the ankles. Lifting or swinging the arms up over the head gets the heart rate up much faster and burns more calories. You can increase these weights as you get used to them. **This is an easy, effective and inexpensive way to tone muscles.**

Once you have mastered one exercise, you can step up to a higher activity level exercise. Read over the list to see which ones burn more calories, and find one you truly enjoy. Once you have achieved your ideal weight, continue the exercise routine, or even step up a level, to maintain optimal good health and the ideal weight.

Easy Weight Loss Secrets

Try these tips for fast and easy weight loss. Step on the scale a week later, or a month later and be amazed at the results. Be sure to also follow the Healthy Diet Basics outlined earlier.

- Many of your favorite foods come in low calorie, light, sugar free, low fat, and fat free versions that taste great. Try several until you find some you like. The result of switching to the low calorie versions of foods and drinks is fast and easy weight loss. Try switching for ¼ or ½ of the foods and beverages you consume, and be amazed at the results.

- Do splurge occasionally and do include your favorite foods in your lifetime weight management plan. Everyone wants to enjoy special foods and drinks for holidays, special occasions, eating out with friends, and just because it's good to treat yourself.

- Remember that almost everything is good for you IN MODERATION! Even a chocolate bar has some health benefits. Enjoy what you love in moderation, and don't let excess destroy your diet.

- After the special occasions, you can easily get right back into the pattern of healthy eating. Many successful dieters occasionally skip the meat dish or the side dish, and instead enjoy the dessert or other favorites. This is a guilt-free option that won't be hard to work off.

- By switching to the sugar free or calorie-free version of most of your beverages, you can cut your daily caloric intake considerably; even up to 800 calories per day, with very little effort.

- When you choose foods in the low calorie, light, sugar free, low fat, or fat free versions, you save anywhere from 10% to 90% of the calories for that dish. For example, a rice dish made with 1 tablespoon of regular butter has 250 calories. If you use fat free margarine instead of regular butter, the total calories are about 150, saving you 100 calories. A salad with 2 tablespoons of fat free dressing instead of regular dressing saves you about 120 calories.

- Prepare your food without adding cooking oil that has 120 calories per tablespoon. Try baking, broiling, or grilling with a non-stick cooking spray that has zero calories.

- With sugar free fruit flavored beverages like *Crystal Light* or *Kool Aid*, you can save about 100 calories per cup over regular fruit flavored beverages. These come in many varieties and are excellent thirst quenchers. With soft drinks, you can reduce the calories from about 150 to zero by switching to a diet version of the soda.

- For between meal snacks, try anything low calorie, and low fat. Some examples are sugar free gum and candy, vegetables with fat free dip, carrot sticks, pretzels, crackers, and any diet beverage. With just a small snack you will easily be able to curb your cravings for an hour or two until your next meal.

- **Choose foods that are low in fat, salt, and sugar. These foods are naturally lower in calories and promote weight loss.** High fat diets have multiple detrimental effects to your health in addition to weight gain. Also avoid high sodium foods to avoid water retention weight gain. Sodium or salt intake should be minimized. High sodium diets can detrimentally affect your entire cardiovascular system, including your heart, and can detrimentally increase your blood pressure. Most processed foods and restaurant foods are high in sodium already, so there is no need to add salt. Try adding just a bit of pepper instead. When eating at home, try to switch to a salt-free substitute, or, if this is too bland, then try to use a mixture of ½ salt, and ½ salt substitute. This substitute of ½ each is healthier, lowers your salt intake, and also tastes great! Add a dash of pepper on top or a dash of cayenne powder to spice it up. **Also, when shopping, look at generic store brands which are almost always lower in calories, salt/sodium, and fat than name-brand foods, and many of these taste great.**

- Many successful dieters take a multi-vitamin/mineral supplement every day including a calcium supplement. (Many vitamins do not supply the recommended daily amount of calcium.) They also take herbal supplements including a daily fruit and vegetable tablet, and a daily apple cider vinegar plus green tea supplement. These herbal supplements provide a variety of health benefits, and some claim they can help promote weight loss. Also, if you are unable to get all the fruits and vegetables in your diet every day, this will be a good replacement with near zero calories. Take these with meals and be sure to drink 6-8 glasses of water daily.

- **Add a little physical activity at least three to five days per week.** Read the fitness guide which includes calorie expenditure charts as related to exercise. To begin, choose a simple and pleasant exercise such as walking, swimming, or riding a bicycle. Just 20 minutes per day, a few days per week, can dramatically accelerate your weight loss, increase energy levels, and improve your overall sense of well being. Your brain releases endorphins when you exercise. Endorphins are chemicals that make you feel good, and the feeling can last for many hours after you finish exercising. Many people who exercise regularly say they feel energized all day long.

Please Note: As with any weight management plan, results may vary for each individual. You should always consult your physician before beginning any new diet or exercise plan; and especially if you have current health problems, or you are pregnant or nursing. This diet plan is offered only as information, for use in maintaining and promoting good health. In the event that the information presented in this diet plan is used without a physician's approval, the individual using the plan accepts all responsibility. This plan is only intended for healthy adults over age 18. Always consult your physician first.

Ideal Body Weight Chart

The following chart is to help calculate ideal body weight for adults. The data is compiled from various health journals. There is a wide range of what is considered to be the "ideal" body weight. This chart lists weights for a medium frame, with one to two pounds of clothing on. Heights listed are without shoes. It is best to weigh yourself in the morning, before eating or drinking anything. This is the best way to track the trend of your weight loss. Weight can fluctuate throughout the day, especially after eating a meal. Use this chart only as an estimated guide to your ideal weight.

FEMALE:

Height (Feet' Inches")	Ideal Body Weight (in Pounds)
5'0"	100 – 110
5'1"	102 – 112
5'2"	105 – 118
5'3"	108 – 122
5'4"	110 – 125
5"5"	114 – 130
5'6"	116 – 136
5'7"	120 – 140
5'8"	125 – 145
5'10"	130 – 155

MALE:

Height (Feet' Inches")	Ideal Body Weight (in Pounds)
5'4"	125 – 140
5'6"	135 – 155
5'8"	145 – 165
5'10"	160 – 175
6'0"	170 – 185
6'2"	180 – 195

Let's face it, we all want to be lean and toned while not having to put in extraordinary effort. This book gives you all the secrets to safe, easy, effective, and permanent results in managing your weight. You can enjoy a lifetime of optimal health at your perfect weight. Inside, find the power and the knowledge to control your weight forever. No fad diets or extreme maneuvers are going to work for long. We all need permanent and easy-to-follow solutions to stay physically fit.

First, you need a fast & easy to use calorie counter to help you make smart food choices. Whether you are a pro, or a novice at counting calories, you will find this book contains the data you need for fast, easy, accurate calorie counts. Experts agree calories count first in weight management. The EASY Lifetime Diet & Exercise Guide is included to help you lose weight faster, and shape and tone your body, while achieving optimal health. Included is information about understanding calories, understanding calorie expenditure, lifestyle activity factors, and simple tips for achieving your goals. This book contains the essential tools for easy lifetime weight management.

Inside find all the foods you love to eat. All the most popular and most common foods, fast food restaurants, brand names, beverages, and alcohol. About 3,500 listings included. This book is available in ebook for download or print edition. Also available from this author is the "Easy Calorie, Carb, Fat, Fiber & Protein Counter".

NOTES

Made in the USA
Monee, IL
19 August 2021

76110294R00069